OXFORD MEDICAL PUBLICATIONS

Cachexia–Anorexia in Cancer Patients

Cachexia–Anorexia in Cancer Patients

Edited by

Eduardo Bruera

*Edmonton General Hospital
Edmonton, Canada*

and

Irene Higginson

*London School of Hygiene and
Tropical Medicine, London, UK*

Toronto

PRESS

1996

Oxford University Press, Walton Street, Oxford OX2 6DP

Oxford   New York

Athens   Auckland   Bangkok   Bombay
Calcutta   Cape Town   Dar es Salaam   Delhi
Florence   Hong Kong   Istanbul   Karachi
Kuala Lumpur   Madras   Madrid   Melbourne
Mexico City   Nairobi   Paris   Singapore
Taipei   Tokyo   Toronto
and associated companies in
Berlin   Ibadan

Oxford is a trade mark of Oxford University Press

Published in the United States
by Oxford University Press Inc., New York

© E. Bruera, I. Higginson and the contributors listed on pp. ix–x, 1996

A catalogue record for this book is available from the British Library

Library of Congress Cataloging in Publication Data
Cachexia–anorexia in cancer patients / edited by Eduardo Bruera and Irene Higginson
(Oxford medical publications)
Includes bibliographical references and index.
1. Cancer–Nutritional aspects.   2. Cachexia.   3. Anorexia.
4. Cancer–complications.   I. Bruera, Eduardo.   II. Higginson, Irene.   III. Series.
[DNLM: 1. Cachexia–etiology.   2. Cachexia–therapy.   3. Anorexia–therapy
4. Neoplasms–complications. WB 146 C119 1996]
RC268.45.C33 1996   616.99'4–dc20   96-1506
ISBN 0 19 262540 3

Typeset by Hewer Text Composition Services, Edinburgh

Printed in Great Britain by Bookcraft (Bath) Ltd, Midsomer Norton, Avon

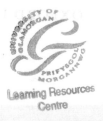

Preface

Cancer is one of the most frequent causes of death in both developed and developing countries. The current situation is likely to become worse in the future since the mortality rates of the five most frequent cancers have not changed significantly in the last 20 years, the age-corrected mortality of frequent cancers such as those of the lung and colon is increasing, and there is a generalized ageing of the population.

The vast majority of patients who die of advanced cancer present with a combination of anorexia, cachexia, asthenia, and chronic nausea. This extremely complex and frequent syndrome has been recently referred to as the 'cachexia–anorexia syndrome'. This syndrome, together with cancer pain, is one of the two most frequent and devastating problems that affect patients with advanced and terminal cancer. However, while significant literature and comprehensive books have been written on the management of cancer pain, there is a limited amount of comprehensive literature on the management of the cachexia–anorexia syndrome. Moreover, most of the monographs and reviews on this subject have been limited to narrow aspects of the problem such as the pathophysiology of cachexia or the effects of total parenteral nutrition on cachexia. Therefore, a comprehensive review of basic and clinical aspects of the cachexia–anorexia syndrome is lacking.

We believe that such a review is particularly appropriate at the present moment. Following several years of limited developments, during the last 5 years there has been significant improvement in our understanding of the pathophysiology of cancer cachexia. Clinicians should be aware of these developments because they either have already or will soon have direct diagnostic and therapeutic implications.

In the area of clinical evaluation of cancer patients there has been an increasing emphasis on the assessment and management of symptoms, physical function, and overall quality of life. Cachexia has a major impact on these three areas and its effects should be reviewed accordingly.

Finally, in the area of therapeutics, agents have emerged during recent years that might have significant effects on the clinical course of anorexia and cachexia.

Cachexia–anorexia should no longer be accepted as a 'normal' manifestation of advanced cancer that requires no further assessment or treatment. Our book attempts to present the reader with a strategy for an evidence-based approach to this syndrome in his or her patients. This book is addressed primarily to physicians with an interest in the clinical management of cancer patients. This includes specialists in medical, radiation and surgical oncology, and palliative medicine, as well as general physicians and family doctors, many of whom care for patients with cancer. We hope that clinical researchers will also find value in the appraisals of research evidence and the highlighting of areas which remain under-researched.

We hope that the readers will gain an understanding of the magnitude and complexity of the problem of cachexia–anorexia in cancer, including the known and postulated mechanisms for aetiology, the impact on the patient and family, and the process of assessment and ethical decision-making regarding management of this devastating syndrome.

Edmonton and London   E. B.
1996   I. H.

Contents

Contributors

Dr H. Richard Alexander
Metabolism Section, Surgery Branch, National Cancer Institute, National Institutes of Health Building 10, Room 2B17, Bethesda, MD 20892, USA.

Dr Kevin G. Billingsley
Metabolism Section, Surgery Branch, National Cancer Institute, National Institutes of Health Building 10, Room 2B17, Bethesda, MD 20892, USA.

Dr Eduardo Bruera
Palliative Care Program, Edmonton General Hospital, 11111 Jasper Avenue, Edmonton, Alberta, Canada T5K 0L4.

Dr Rachel Burman
Trinity Hospice, 30 Clapham Common North Side, London SW4 0RN, UK.

Dr Joe Chamberlain
Trinity Hospice, 30 Clapham Common North Side, London SW4 0RN, UK.

Franco De Conno
Pain Therapy and Palliative Care Division, National Cancer Institute, via Venezian 1, 20133 Milan, Italy.

Dr Robert Dunlop
St Christopher's Hospice, 51 Lawrie Park Road, Sydenham, London SE26 6DZ, UK.

Dr Robin Fainsinger
Palliative Care Program, Edmonton General Hospital, 11111 Jasper Avenue, Edmonton, Alberta, Canada T5K 0L4.

Dr Brett T. Gemlo
Department of Surgery, Division of Colon and Rectal Surgery, University of Minneapolis, Minneapolis, MN, USA.

Dr Irene Higginson
Health Services Research Unit, London School of Hygiene and Tropical Medicine, Keppel Street, London WC1, UK.

Dr Jane Ingham
Department of Neurology, Memorial Sloan–Kettering Cancer Center, 1275 York Avenue, New York, NY 10021, USA.

Dr Neil MacDonald
Center for Bioethics, Clinical Research Institute of Montreal, 110 Pine Avenue West, Montreal, Quebec, Canada H2W 1R7.

Dr Hans Neuenschwander
Hospice Lugano and Department of Oncology, Ticino, Switzerland.

Dr Jose Pereira
Palliative Care Program, Edmonton General Hospital, 11111 Jasper Avenue, Edmonton, Alberta, Canada T5K 0L4.

Dr Russell Portenoy
Department of Neurology, Memorial Sloan–Kettering Cancer Center, 1275 York Avenue, New York, NY 10021, USA.

Dr Carla Ripamonti
Pain Therapy and Palliative Care Division, National Cancer Institute, via Venezian 1, 20133 Milan, Italy.

Alberto Sbanotto
Pain Therapy and Palliative Care, European Institute of Oncology, Milan, Italy.

Dr Antonio Vigano
Palliative Care Program, Edmonton General Hospital, 11111 Jasper Avenue, Edmonton, Alberta, Canada T5K 0L4.

Catherine Winget
Centre for the Economics of Mental Health, Institute of Psychiatry, De Crespigny Park, Denmark Hill, London SE5, UK.

The pathophysiology of cachexia in advanced cancer and AIDS

Kevin G. Billingsley and H. Richard Alexander

INTRODUCTION

In recent years developments in molecular biology techniques have provided a rapidly expanding body of knowledge about the possible cellular mechanisms which mediate cancer cachexia and the response of the host to neoplastic disease. In spite of this burgeoning knowledge base, cachexia remains a clinically significant problem in cancer patients, but also in the increasingly large group of patients with acquired immune deficiency syndrome (AIDS). Although the prevalence of cachexia varies with the type of malignancy and the sensitivity of the nutritional assessment methods used, significant nutritional compromise affects 50–80% of patients with neoplastic disease, (1) (see Chapter 6). In fact, cancer cachexia is implicated as a major factor in the ultimate demise of the individual in up to 50% of all cancer patients. (2–4) A similar type of profound protein calorie malnutrition also appears to affect the majority of AIDS patients in the later stages of illness. (5–8) Like patients with malignant disease, AIDS patients are devastated by the debilitating effects of cachexia. Weight loss generally occurs early in the course of the disease and increases in severity with disease progression. (9) In cancer patients, nutritional deterioration impacts negatively on the patient's ability to respond to antineoplastic therapy, as well as their overall survival. In the majority of tumor types, stage for stage median survival was significantly shorter in patients who had experienced significant weight loss prior to initiating therapy (10) (Table 1.1). Antineoplastic therapies, including surgery, chemotherapy, radiation therapy, and immunotherapy, have made strides forward in recent years. However, patients who are debilitated by cachexia frequently cannot tolerate these therapeutic interventions and they suffer from increased morbidity of cancer treatment. For AIDS patients, the profound protein calorie malnutrition of the cachectic syndrome appears to contribute significantly to the progressive immunocompromise of human immunodeficiency virus (HIV) infection.

A major area of recent investigation is the study of the function of cytokines and other soluble mediators in the pathophysiology of cancer cachexia. Tumor necrosis factor (TNF)/cachectin appears likely to play a role both in humans and in animal models. Administration of recombinant TNF to animals reproduces the weight loss and many of the metabolic alterations observed in cancer cachexia. (11, 12) Detectable levels of TNF are present in the serum of some patients with cancer and AIDS, (13) although other studies demonstrate that TNF cannot uniformly be detected in serum and suggest that it may exert its effects at a local or tissue level. (14, 15)

Table 1.1 Frequency of weight loss, relationship to performance status, and impact on survival in patients, undergoing chemotherapy for advanced commonly diagnosed cancers

Diagnosis	n	% with weight loss in prior 6 months	% with weight loss and normal performance	Survival (weeks) of patients with and without weight loss		% decrease in survival with weight loss
				with	without	
Lung, non-small cell	590	61	56	20	14	30*
Lung, small cell	436	57	47	34	27	21*
Colon	307	54	45	43	21	51*
Breast	289	36	25	70	45	36*
Prostate	78	56	35	46	24	48*
Gastric, non–measurable	179	83	80	41	27	34*
Gastric measurable	138	87	86	18	16	11
Pancreas	111	83	78	14	12	14

* $p < 0.05$.
Table abstracted from DeWys and others, Am. J. Med. 1980;69 491–9 (1).

Recent studies demonstrate potential roles for multiple additional cytokines including interleukin-1 (IL–1), interleukin-6 (IL–6), Interferon gamma (IFN–γ) and leukemia inhibitory factor. Because the cachectic syndrome is most likely the result of a complex orchestration of signaling molecules, no single dominant mediator is likely to emerge. However, the availability of anticytokine antibodies and increasingly sophisticated molecular biology techniques will most likely provide a more detailed understanding of complex cytokine pathways in the near future.

CLINICAL FEATURES OF CACHEXIA

Although there is a broad spectrum of clinical presentation, almost all patients suffering from cachexia exhibit a constellation of weight loss, anorexia, weakness, and inanition. This clinical picture results primarily from progressive wasting of structural protein and energy stores. This wasting inevitably leads to a global functional decline of the host. The underlying perturbations in host carbohydrate, lipid, and protein metabolism are manifested in a variety of laboratory abnormalities. Cachectic individuals demonstrate measurable degrees of hypertriglyceridemia, hypoalbuminemia, hypoproteinemia, anemia, glucose intolerance, and lactic acidosis.

In cancer-bearing patients, different malignant histologies appear to produce varying degrees of cachectic change. Patients with cancer of the esophagus, cardia, stomach, pancreas, and small cell carcinoma of the lung frequently have the most profound weight loss at initial presentation. Conversely, early weight loss is relatively unusual in patients with testicular cancer, sarcoma, breast cancer, and ovarian cancer. (16)

Similar to cancer patients, AIDS patients also develop a syndrome of progressive weight loss with erosion of host adipose tissue and muscle mass. The Centers for Disease Control has indicated that wasting with constitutional symptoms of more than 30 days' duration and the presence of the antibody against HIV are sufficient to make the diagnosis of AIDS, even in the absence of opportunistic infection or malignancy. (17) As in the case of malignant disease, anorexia is a central feature of HIV-related wasting. Multiple factors impact on declining caloric intake. AIDS patients suffer from a variety of gastrointestinal pathologies which impair their food intake and nutrient absorption. Such pathology ranges from candidal or herpetic infection of the upper aerodigestive tract to chronic diarrhea related to intestinal infection of a host by pathogenic organisms.

The anorexia of the cachexia syndrome is a relative hypophagia. Cachectic individuals suffer from a progressive diminution in nutrient intake such that energy intake falls short of metabolic requirements. When a negative energy balance results there is a loss of lipid and protein stores. The etiology of this anorexia appears to be multifactorial (Fig. 1.1). Multiple endogenous mediators are produced by both the tumor and the host. In tumor-bearing animal models, cytokines such as TNF, IL–1, and IFN–γ appear to contribute directly to anorexia. (18–20) In addition, there are multiple treatment-related effects which impact on nutrient intake. Chemotherapy and radiation therapy both produce varying degrees of nausea, vomiting, and mucositis. (21) When therapy-related nausea and vomiting occur in close proximity to oral intake, patients frequently develop learned food aversions. These learned aversions also extend to anticipatory nausea and vomiting. These symptoms can be so severe that patients have difficulty tolerating certain foods, even weeks after therapy has ceased. (22) There is also evidence that many chemotherapeutic regimens produce altered taste perceptions such that once-desirable meals become virtually unpalatable. (23)

Some malignancies result in mechanical disruptions of alimentation. This is clearly the case with squamous cell tumors of the head, neck, and esophagus. Gastric, pancreatic, and colon tumors can also cause intraluminal gastrointestinal tract obstruction. In these cases, surgical resection or bypass of the obstructed segment may greatly improve the hypophagia.

In some cancer patients, impairment of nutrient intake and digestion is functional rather than mechanical. Chronic nausea in patients with advanced cancer is sometimes related to a syndrome of autonomic insufficiency. This type of autonomic failure can cause markedly impaired gastric emptying and gastric stasis. (24) This syndrome is most prevalent in disseminated intra-abdominal malignancies, but a component of autonomic failure may be an under-appreciated contributor to the nausea and anorexia of many patients with advanced cancer.

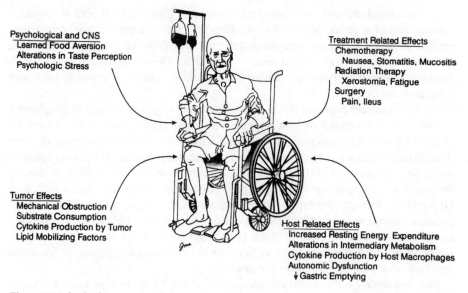

Psychological and CNS
  Learned Food Aversion
  Alterations in Taste Perception
  Psychologic Stress

Treatment Related Effects
  Chemotherapy
    Nausea, Stomatitis, Mucositis
  Radiation Therapy
    Xerostomia, Fatigue
  Surgery
    Pain, Ileus

Tumor Effects
  Mechanical Obstruction
  Substrate Consumption
  Cytokine Production by Tumor
  Lipid Mobilizing Factors

Host Related Effects
  Increased Resting Energy Expenditure
  Alterations in Intermediary Metabolism
  Cytokine Production by Host Macrophages
  Autonomic Dysfunction
  ↓ Gastric Emptying

Fig. 1.1 Multiple factors contribute to the anorexia and wasting of the clinical syndrome of cancer cachexia.

ALTERED METABOLISM IN CACHEXIA

One of the principal early observations in the study of a cancer cachexia was the finding by Cori and Cori (25) that the venous effluent from a sarcoma-bearing chick wing had decreased concentrations of glucose and elevated levels of lactate when compared to the contralateral non-tumor-bearing wing. This observation suggested that the sarcoma was utilizing glucose and producing large amounts of lactic acid. This type of tumor avidity for metabolic substrate led many subsequent investigators to theorize that the progressive wasting of cachexia resulted from the ability of neoplastic tissue to sequester metabolic fuels at the expense of the host metabolism. In reality, however, the situation is more complex than a simple loss of substrate to tumor metabolism. The weight of current evidence suggests multiple alterations in host intermediary metabolism result from the effects of a number of circulating factors. These factors appear to be released not only by the tumor itself, but also by the host organism in response to the tumor. Several lines of evidence support this notion. In many cases, alterations in host metabolism in cancer patients can be measured in the presence of a very small tumor burden and tumor weight at autopsy rarely exceeds 5% of host body weight. Thus, it is unlikely that the changes of cachexia are caused merely by consumption of substrate by tumor. Further, a number of specific metabolic changes can be detected in the host at sites remote from the tumor.

ENERGY EXPENDITURE

The cachectic syndrome exhibited by both AIDS and cancer patients demonstrates numerous metabolic perturbations involving overall energy expenditure as well as alterations in glucose, protein, and lipid metabolism. These changes are unlike the metabolism of starvation and are more closely related to the metabolic picture of severe trauma and sepsis. (25) This concept is evident in the fact that cachectic patients will continue to lose weight even when aggressive nutritional supplementation is used to provide adequate caloric intake. In one study, head and neck cancer patients were fed via continuous enteral alimentation under metabolic ward conditions and failed to gain significant quantities of weight. (27) Nutritional supplementation has also been considered in the form of total parenteral nutrition (TPN) (29–30; and see Chapter 9).

Evidence exists which indicates that the overall metabolic rate is increased in the cachectic host. Hyltander *et al.* (31) examined the resting energy expenditure (REE) in 106 cancer patients and 96 non-cancer-bearing controls. The cancer patients had an elevated REE compared to both weight-losing and weight-stable control patients. (31) Despite these perceived differences, other investigators have demonstrated that measured differences in the levels of the REE are abolished when levels are corrected for measurements of lean body mass. (32) In a study of patients with non-metastatic primary sarcomas, REE was significantly higher in the sarcoma patients than in the controls, even when corrected for lead body mass. (33) Differences also appear to exist between different types of malignancies. Studies of patients with small cell lung cancer have an increased REE compared to healthy controls, but patients with colon cancer demonstrate no significant differences from controls. (34) This pattern of elevated energy expenditure in the face of anorexia and diminished caloric intake is one of the key features which distinguishes the cachectic syndrome from starvation alone. Healthy individuals when confronted with reduced caloric consumption adapt their metabolic profile so that the overall energy expenditure is diminished. Body lipids become the preferential metabolic substrate, with relative preservation of lean muscle until late in the course of starvation. In a manner similar to cancer patients, individuals with AIDS also demonstrate an elevated metabolic rate with an elevated REE. (35, 36) It is not clear to what extent this alteration is due to primary HIV infection versus the effects of the multiple, sometimes occult, opportunistic infections which plague these patients.

CARBOHYDRATE METABOLISM

Alteration in carbohydrate metabolism is one of the most common clinical features observed in cachectic patients. Multiple studies have demonstrated that neoplastic tissue uses glucose preferentially and relies heavily on the glycolytic pathway for energy production. (37, 38) This may be due to basic mechanisms of tumor metabolism or may simply reflect the fact that much neoplastic tissue survives on marginal oxygenation due to poor tumor vascularity. This in turn necessitates anaerobic metabolism.

The most significant components of altered carbohydrate metabolism appear, however, to be related to host factors rather than tumor metabolism. Experimental animal studies provide the opportunity of measuring glucose metabolism in an untreated, reproducible model of a tumor-bearing host. The effects of simple starvation and decreased food intake can be examined by the use of pair-fed controls. It is critical, however, to bear in mind the inherent limitations of these studies. Most rodent models of cancer cachexia involve a tumor mass which grows to 20–30% of the animal's weight. This tumor mass relative to body weight is rarely seen in human patients. In animal models using massive tumor burdens it has become evident that a portion of the metabolic derangements observed are created by the physical mass of the tumor alone and have little to do with the neoplastic character of the mass. (39) This has been demonstrated by implanting animals with inert, artificial tumors. The mass of these artificial tumors increased the REE up to 11% in these animals. Although these metabolic changes are less pronounced than in an equivalent tumor-bearing state, it demonstrates one of the limitations of using rodent tumor models to study cachexia.

An early observation which was made in experimental animals and then subsequently in humans is that there is almost always a marked increase in hepatic glucose production in the cachectic host. In tumor-bearing rats, radiolabeled tracer studies show increased rates of hepatic gluconeogenesis. This carbon flux through the Cori cycle involves mobilization of peripheral protein stores which provides amino acid substrate, particularly alanine and glutamine, for gluconeogenesis. Increased Cori cycle activity also relies on a supply of lactate for conversion back into glucose. Lactate is supplied by the increased glycolytic activity of both the tumor and host. Glucose in turn is converted back to lactate by glycolysis. Such 'futile cycling' is metabolically inefficient and may account for up to 300 kcal/day in energy loss. (40)

Cachectic animals demonstrate hepatocellular adaptations to support increased gluconeogenesis. The activity of gluconeogenic enzymes including glucose-6-phosphatase and phosphoenolpyruvate carboxykinase (PEP) are elevated in tumor-bearing animals. This elevation does not appear to be secondary to elevated insulin levels which increase only minimally in cachectic tumor-bearing animals. (41)

When hepatic glucose production is measured in humans, the picture is more difficult to interpret. Most studies have been performed in a heterogeneous group of patients with a wide range of ages, nutritional characteristics, and varying histories of antineoplastic therapy. An additional confounding difficulty is the need for non-cancer-bearing, weight-losing individuals to serve as appropriate controls. In spite of these limitations, some consistent features have emerged. As observed in experimental models, cancer patients consistently demonstrate increased rates of hepatic gluconeogenesis and carbon recycling. In patients with extremity sarcomas, glucose uptake is higher in the tumor-bearing limb than in the contralateral control limb. (42) Patients with localized esophageal cancer demonstrate elevated levels of glucose turnover in forearm muscle. (43) Although the findings of these two studies are similar, they point to different mechanisms creating alterations in carbohydrate metabolism. The increased glucose uptake within sarcoma-bearing limbs suggests that increased glucose demand by a tumor is a significant component in disordered carbohydrate metabolism. The changes observed in the patients with esophageal carcinoma indicate that the cachectic state involves a global increase in host metabolism, not merely an increase in metabolic demand by the tumor itself. In reality, both mechanisms are likely to contribute to clinical cachexia.

Circulating lactate levels are also increased in tumor-bearing individuals. (44, 45) Elevated lactate appears to be primarily related to the preference of neoplastic tissue for anaerobic metabolism, but skeletal muscle may also serve as a lactate source. (46)

Some investigators have attempted to quantify lactate in venous effluent from tumors. In an evaluation of head and neck tumors by Richtsmeier, *et al.*, there was a significant release of lactate into the tumor-draining vein. Similar observations have been made in lung cancer patients when lactate levels are measured in draining veins from the involved portion of the lung. (48)

Another common finding is that cancer-bearing hosts have a significant degree of glucose intolerance. (49) Physiologically, this glucose intolerance replicates type II diabetes mellitus. Patients are neither insulinopenic nor do they develop ketoacidosis. The picture is rather one of marked insulin resistance. Glicksman and Rawson (50) evaluated over 600 cancer patients and demonstrated that approximately 37% have diabetic glucose tolerance curves. Patients with sarcomas also have abnormal glucose tolerance profiles, even before the development of cachexia. (52) The insulin resistance seen in cachectic patients has several manifestations. As described, insulin resistance at the hepatocellular level is expressed as increased glucose recycling via gluconeogenesis. At the periphery, the ability of skeletal muscle to take up glucose is limited both in the fasting state as well as in the fed state characterized by insulin abundance. (52) The ability of skeletal muscle to process glucose into glycogen is also significantly compromised. (53) Unlike diabetic patients, however, cachectic individuals do not demonstrate marked increases in circulating insulin levels. (54)

LIPID METABOLISM

The clinical *sine qua non* of the cachectic syndrome is loss of host adipose tissue. There are a number of significant alterations in lipid metabolism which underlie this loss of body fat. Lipid is an important fuel source that provides a significant percentage of the metabolic substrate which is necessary to support the elevated REE observed in the cachectic syndrome. Animal models demonstrate elevated levels of circulating triglycerides as well as non-essential fatty acids. (55) Increased plasma levels of triglycerides appear to be related to decreased activity of the enzyme lipoprotein lipase. This enzyme facilitates hydrolysis of chylomicrons and low-density lipoprotein triglycerides to fatty acids. Free fatty acids can in turn by taken up by adipocytes and coupled with glycerol in triglyceride synthesis. Down-regulation of lipoprotein lipase activity appears to be one of the common pathways by which multiple cachectic mediators exert their effects. This down-regulation significantly diminishes the process of lipogenesis. Investigators have also studied the possibility that the cachectic host suffers from increased levels of lipolysis as well as decreased lipogenesis. Evaluations of host glycerol turnover and clearance have yielded conflicting results about the role of lipolytic activity in cachexia. In one study of patients with documented weight loss, elevated rates of plasma glycerol turnover pointed towards an increased rate of whole body lipolysis. (56) Using a similar method of glycerol turnover analysis, Jeevanandam *et al.* (62) have shown that the rates of lipolysis in nine cancer-bearing patients were not significantly different from those observed in five control patients. However, glycerol clearance, which reflects lipogenesis, was significantly less in cancer patients relative to the controls. (57) When a group of cachectic patients with esophageal cancer were compared to nutritionally matched control groups both with and without cancer, elevated rates of lipolytic activity appeared to be correlated with a nutritional deficit, not with the cancer-bearing state *per se*. (43) In summary, hypertriglyceridemia, with significant lipid wasting, is a common metabolic motif in cachectic patients. A component of the lipid loss observed in these patients appears to be related to their nutritionally depleted state resulting from anorexia and hypophagia, but an equally significant portion of adipose loss stems from fundamental changes in lipid metabolism, principally inhibition of lipoprotein lipase activity.

Like cancer patients, a significant number of individuals with AIDS develop measurable hypertriglyceridemia during their clinical course. In a group of patients who had their body composition and triglycerides measured, 50% demonstrated hypertriglyceridemia. (52) However, there was no relationship between increased serum triglycerides and clinical wasting.

PROTEIN METABOLISM

Although loss of host adipose tissue comprises much of the weight loss in cancer cachexia, protein catabolism and skeletal muscle breakdown probably account for a great deal of the morbidity. Protein metabolism has been studied in both experimental animals and human patients. Animal studies offer the advantages of precisely regulated experimental conditions and the use of pair-fed animals to control for the effects of nutritional depletion in the non-tumor-bearing state. As discussed, however, these studies are frequently limited by reliance on inordinately large tumor burdens to produce measurable cachectic changes. Acknowledging the limitations of such animal models, these studies have nevertheless provided a number of insights into protein metabolism in the tumor-bearing state.

Mice bearing the MAC 16 adenocarcinoma undergo a 60% decline in protein synthesis and increased protein degradation when they have lost 15–30% of their body weight. Serum from these cachectic animals has proteolytic activity when applied to an isolated gastrocnemius muscle *in vitro*. This suggests a soluble proteolytic factor is present in the serum of these animals. (58)

Amino acids released from skeletal muscle in cachectic animals serve as the primary substrate for gluconeogenesis. When phosphenol pyruvate carboxykinase, the rate-limiting enzyme of hepatic gluconeogenesis, is inhibited by hydrazine, plasma amino acid levels increase significantly more in tumor-bearing animals than in controls. (59) There is also evidence that the rate of conversion from alanine to glucose is increased in the tumor-bearing animal. (41, 60)

Although studies of protein metabolism in human patients clearly provide valuable clinical information, they have their own set of methodological shortcomings. Techniques of clinical evaluation such as history, physical examination, and anthropometry provide limited, overall assessments of protein metabolism in large groups of patients. Research methods such as nitrogen balance studies and labeled amino acid kinetics provide detailed metabolic information about a limited number of patients. These studies are also hampered by the limited availability of appropriate non-cancer-bearing control patients. A non-cancer-bearing group is particularly difficult to accrue because relatively few non-malignant diseases in the elderly are associated with progressive weight loss.

In spite of these limitations, several consistent features have emerged from clinical studies. Most studies of whole-body amino acid kinetics demonstrate increased rates of whole-body amino acid turnover, with increased hepatic protein synthesis and catabolism of skeletal muscle proteins in both weight-losing and weight-stable cancer patients. (61–64) In many ways the pattern of protein metabolism in the cachectic host replicates the protein metabolism of patients in the catabolic phase of sepsis or trauma. The overall increase in protein turnover arises from the release of significant quantities of amino acids from peripheral muscle stores with a concomitant increase in hepatic protein synthesis and gluconeogenesis. Hepatocytes isolated from patients with malignancy show an increase in protein synthesis compared to patients with benign disease. (65) These appear to be primarily acute phase reactants such as C-reactive protein, γ-1-antitrypsin and haptoglobin. Hepatic synthesis of functional proteins, such as albumin and transferrin is, however, decreased in cachectic conditions. (66) Further, skeletal muscle from cancer-bearing patients demonstrates increased protein degradation and decreased protein synthesis. (67)

Investigations of protein metabolism in AIDS patients reveal equivocal findings. In one study, protein loss was not found to be accelerated in AIDS patients. (68) However, nitrogen balance surveys indicate that the majority of AIDS patients have a significant negative nitrogen balance. (69)

MECHANISMS OF CANCER CACHEXIA

A number of studies provide evidence for an array of soluble mediators which produce the changes in intermediary metabolism that lead to the wasting of cachexia. Norton *et al.* (70) performed a series of experiments with rats using paired animals with a surgically created parabiotic anastomosis. In these animals a vascular anastamosis was fashioned such that they had a shared circulation. Only one of these animals had a tumor, yet both animals developed cachectic changes. Each animal, however, was less severely affected than single animals which had matched tumor burdens. These findings argue for the existence of a soluble factor or factors which are capable of traveling to both parabiotes and can mediate the metabolic changes of cachexia. A similar conclusion can be made from the experiments of Illig *et al.* (71) These investigators harvested serum from both tumor-bearing and control rats. They subsequently treated naïve rats with the serum. Rats treated with regular doses of serum from tumor-bearing animals developed profound cachexia. Rats treated with control serum were unaffected. In humans, clinicians have repeatedly observed that cachexia often arises relatively early in the course of neoplastic disease. It is possible to document multiple changes in intermediary metabolism even with small tumors. This observation provides further indication of the production of soluble mediators producing cachectic changes even when the tumor is too small to cause any local or mass effects. It is not clear from these observations if such a circulating factor is derived from the tumor itself or if it is produced by the host organism in response to a tumor. In all likelihood, production of such mediating factors relies on multiple interactions between the tumor and the host defense system.

A diverse series of both *in vivo* and *in vitro* experiments implicate cytokines as some of the prime mediators of cachexia. Cytokines are polypeptide molecules which are produced by macrophages, monocytes, and lymphocytes. They are not stored intracellularly but are synthesized *de novo* in response to a diverse range of stimuli including microbial invasion, trauma, stress, and neoplastic growth. Cytokines mediate a multitude of biologic effects including fever, lymphocyte proliferation and activation, the hepatic acute phase response, and, in some cases, regression of tumors. Cytokines act predominantly through localized paracrine and autocrine interactions, but circulating levels of various cytokines can be detected in animal models as well as some human patients with cancer. In cancer patients these cytokines are primarily produced by host inflammatory cells in response to a tumor, although some tumor cells constituitively produce cytokine products.

TUMOR NECROSIS FACTOR

Although the precise role of each individual cytokine within the broad picture of cachexia is difficult to define, there are specific cytokines which clearly appear to be involved (Table 1.2). TNF is a prime candidate in this regard. An early observation that led to the elucidation of TNF function was the finding that rabbits with trypanosomal infections suffered from profound disturbances of lipid metabolism. Guy (72) first observed that these animals were markedly hyperlipidemic. Subsequent studies demonstrated that the hyperlipidemia was primarily a hypertriglyceridemia. (73) There appeared to be suppression of the enzyme lipoprotein lipase leading to a paradoxical accumulation of lipid in the plasma of these anorectic and cachectic animals. Further study indicated that the hypertriglyceridemia of infection was mediated by a factor which was soluble in plasma. This factor clearly suppressed the activity of lipoprotein lipase (LPL) and could be purified from the supernatant of endotoxin-stimulated macrophages. (74) This factor was named 'cachectin', and when it was eventually sequenced it was found to be the murine homologue of human TNF. (75) Human TNF had been so named because it was observed to induce a hemorrhagic necrosis of tumors during states of infection in the host. (76)

Table 1.2 Metabolic alterations of cytokine mediators and cancer cachexia

Parameters	Food Intake	Body weight	Lipids		Proteins		
			Synthesis	Lipolysis	Synthesis[a]	Skeletal muscle proteolysis	APP
Cachexia	↓	↓	↓	↑	↓	↑	↑
TNF–α	↓	↓	↓↑[a]	↑	↓	↑	↑
IL–1	↓	↓	↓	↑	↓	↑[b]	↑
IL–6	↓	↓	↓	NA	↓	NA	↑
IFN–β	↓	↓	↓	NA	NA	NA	NA
D–factor	NA	↓	↓	NA	NA	NA	↓

[a] TNF increase hepatic lipid synthesis, but decreased triglyceride synthesis.
[b] IL–1 synergizes with TNF to induce skeletal muscle proteolysis.
[c] Includes synthesis of functional hepatic proteins (albumin, transferrin) and/or skeletal muscle protein.
NA not available.
APP acute phase proteins.

The identification of cachectin/TNF ushered in a new era of investigation in the area of cytokine biology. It became clear that a single host-derived mediator may have multiple biologic activities and may play a substantive role in the pathophysiology of many disease states including endotoxic shock and cancer cachexia. Recent advances in research methodology have greatly facilitated cytokine-related investigations. Principally, the use of recombinant DNA technology to produce large quantities of pure cytokines has enabled researchers to use reproducible cytokine doses in animal experiments and has also made possible the use of cytokines as therapeutic agents.

Considerable efforts have been made to demonstrate circulating levels of TNF and other cytokines in the cancer-bearing host. Balkwill *et al.* (13) demonstrated that 50% of 276 fresh serum samples from cancer-bearing patients had measurable TNF. This has been a difficult finding to replicate. A series of patients with small cell carcinoma of the lung uniformly did not have detectable TNF levels. (77) Similar investigations have been undertaken with AIDS patients. One group has noted elevated levels of TNF in AIDS patients; however, there was no relationship between the degree of weight loss and the levels of circulating TNF. (78) Subsequent studies have found no difference between AIDS patients and control patients. (79–81) Considering the role of cytokines as autocrine and paracrine mediators, it should not be surprising that their presence in plasma seems to be evanescent and, in some ways, inconsistent. By exerting most of their functional effects at a local tissue level, they are not accessible to standard immunoassay of serum samples. One feasible hypothesis is that host macrophages and inflammatory cells are activated within the milieu of the tumor. These cells subsequently migrate to distant locations in the body. At these sites they may exert a potent regulatory effect on host metabolism without releasing substantial quantities of cytokines into the free circulation.

When exogenous TNF is administered to animals, the physiologic effects depend on the dose, route, and timing of administration. Animals become tolerant to the anorectic effects of TNF when it is given as intermittent bolus injections. (82) However, animals receiving continuous doses of TNF through a subcutaneously implanted pump develop dose-dependent anorexia, lean body wasting, and death. (83) Similar effects were noted when nude mice were implanted with tumor cells that were transduced with the human TNF gene. The mice developed progressive anorexia, weight loss, lipid depletion, and earlier death than animals implanted with an identical tumor without the TNF gene. (18) If the same TNF-secreting tumor is implanted intracerebrally, the anorectic effects are even more marked, but there is relative preservation of host protein stores, more compatible with chronic starvation. (84)

Multiple studies illustrate the relationship between TNF and the metabolic alterations which characterize cachexia. In addition to its well-described inhibitory effects on LPL, adipocytes themselves respond to TNF by releasing glycerol and eventually becoming lipid depleted. (85) In diabetic rats in which LPL activity is suppressed, the administration of TNF produces a progressive increase in serum triglycerides. In this case, the triglyceride elevation appears to be related to *de novo* lipogenesis in the liver. (86) In humans, TNF produces hyperlipidemia and increased rates of fatty acid turnover and lipolysis. (87)

In addition to lipid metabolism, TNF also mediates multiple derangements in protein metabolism. Efforts to evaluate the role of TNF in protein metabolism within skeletal muscle has demonstrated several findings. When treated with TNF, rats have a clear activation of muscle protein degradation as measured by ^{3}H methyl histidine release. (88) Another study reported that 4–6 hours after an acute administration of either TNF or IL–1 to rats there was a 2–4-fold activation of muscle branched chain keto acid dehydrogenase. (89) This enzyme regulates branched chain amino acid catabolism in skeletal muscle. This finding suggests that TNF may be playing a role not only in the activation of muscle proteolysis but also in increased catabolism of liberated branched chain amino acids. TNF also acts at a hepatocellular level to regulate protein metabolism. Hepatocytes treated with TNF develop increased rates of amino acid uptake, acute phase protein synthesis, and gluconeogenesis. (65, 90) In spite of this increase in synthesis of acute phase reactants, TNF produces a more generalized hypoproteinemia as manifested by decreased levels of serum albumin.

Efforts have been made to block the cachectic effects of TNF either by inducing tolerance with repeated sublethal doses or by treating animals with anti-TNF antibodies. If rats are made tolerant to TNF and subsequently implanted with an MCA sarcoma, they will survive longer and develop fewer cachectic changes than non-TNF-tolerant, tumor-bearing control animals. (11) This effect is observed in spite of similar rates of tumor growth in both groups. When a group of tumor-bearing rats with the Lewis lung adenocarcinoma were treated with neutralizing antibodies to TNF, they had significant preservation of host body lipid and less hypertriglyceridemia relative to control animals. However, antibody treatment did not significantly alter food intake, changes in body weight, or the changes of anemia and hypoalbuminemia. (91) In another study examining the effects of TNF antibody treatment coupled with IL–1 receptor antagonist (IL–1ra), the treatment preserved the body protein composition in tumor-bearing mice. In this study, however, tumor sizes were significantly less in treated animals compared to controls. In this model, TNF and IL–1 appeared to be functioning as growth factors. The attenuation of cachectic parameters was more likely related to a diminished tumor burden more than any specific anticachectic effect. (92)

INTERLEUKIN–1

Like TNF, IL–1 is a peptide cytokine which has broad physiologic effects and plays a key role in the pro-inflammatory cytokine cascade. Previously called leucocyte endogenous mediator or lymphocyte activation factor, IL–1 is produced in response to microbial invasion, tissue injury, and an array of inflammatory processes. (15, 93–95) As implied by the molecule's early descriptions, it plays a critical role in leukocyte activation and proliferation of both B and T lymphocytes; it also serves to stimulate the hepatic acute phase response and is a potent endogenous pyrogen. Like TNF, IL–1 is produced predominantly by monocytes and macrophages and it appears to be capable of acting synergistically with TNF.

In conjunction with its pro-inflammatory role, IL–1 appears to participate in the pathogenesis of cachexia. Administration of exogenous IL–1 causes fever, inflammation, and anorexia. (96, 97) There is evidence that the anorexia is not mediated by IL–1 directly, but by an IL–1-induced production of corticotropin-releasing factor by the hypothalamus. (98) As in the case of TNF, it is difficult to demonstrate reliably elevated circulating levels of IL–1 in tumor-bearing animals. Lonroth *et al.* (99) attempted to document the presence of increased IL–1 and IL–1 mRNA in the tissues of animals with MCG 101 sarcomas. They show that the tumor itself produced both TNF and IL–1. The mRNA for IL–1 was significantly induced in the spleen relative to the control, but not in other organs. Nor were TNF mRNA levels elevated. (99) In a subsequent study, these investigators attempted to block activity of TNF and IL–1 with TNF antibodies and IL–1ra. In this study, the two agents together ameliorate some cachectic changes, but appear to do so with a reduction in tumor growth. (91)

Administration of exogenous IL–1 does have a number of metabolic effects. It does not appear to have any direct effect on muscle catabolism *in vivo* but it does have a synergistic effect when administered with TNF; (100, 101) it also affects hepatic protein metabolism. Like TNF, IL–1 stimulates the synthesis and release of acute phase proteins and causes a down-regulation of albumin and transferrin synthesis. (102, 103) It also inhibits LPL activity and increases plasma levels of triglycerides. (101, 104) In addition to direct actions, TNF and IL–1 are both involved in the stimulus of other cytokines. In a murine tumor model utilizing the colon 26 adenocarcinoma, IL–1 production by host macrophages serves to augment secretion of cytokine products by the tumor cells. These secondary cytokines, particularly IL–6, may be the effector molecules which actually mediate the metabolic changes of cachexia. (105)

INTERLEUKIN–6

Interleukin–6 is another regulatory cytokine which is produced by multiple cell types in response to trauma, infection, or sepsis. Interleukin–6 has been identified in the sera of septic patients (106) and patients with AIDS. (107) Elevated levels of IL–6 have also been identified in animals bearing tumors of various histologies; IL–6 levels in these animals rise in proportion to tumor burden. (108) Interleukin–6 is also involved in a network of cytokine interactions involving TNF, IL–1, and IFN–γ. (93, 95)

Strassmann *et al.* (109) have developed a murine cachexia model utilizing a colon 26 tumor line which constituitively produces low levels of IL–6. Treatment of these animals with IL–6 antibodies effectively blocks the changes of cachexia. (109) These investigators demonstrate that IL–1 production by host macrophages which infiltrate the tumor can effectively upregulate tumor production of IL–6. Treatment with intratumoral injections of IL–1 receptor antagonist interrupts this network and will also block the changes of cachexia. (110) In this model, IL–6 functions as the most potent effector cytokine mediating the metabolic changes of cachexia. Interleukin–1 production by host macrophages is necessary to increase IL–6 production by tumor cells, but IL–1 appears to have few direct effects.

In our laboratory, we have demonstrated a similar set of interactions in a murine sarcoma tumor model. In this system, TNF, rather than IL–1, appears to drive production of IL–6 and anther pluripotent cytokine, LIF, by tumor cells. We believe that this type of interaction is a recurring motif in cytokine biology. Specifically, the cachectic syndrome relies on an interaction between host inflammatory cells and tumors to produce significant quantities of cytokine mediators which act both locally and at distant sites to create the metabolic changes of the cachectic syndrome.

INTERFERON γ

Interferon gamma is a cytokine which is synthesized primarily by activated T lymphocytes. It plays a significant role in host defense against viral infection. Like many of the pro-inflammatory cytokines, IFN has a number of metabolic effects when administered to animals. It down-regulates LPL and decreases the rates of fatty acid synthesis in adipocytes. (111) Administration of anti-IFN antibodies to tumor-bearing rats will improve food intake, ameliorate weight loss, and improve survival. (112) The role of IFN relative to other cytokines in the pathogenesis of the cachectic syndrome remains to be clarified.

LEUKEMIA INHIBITORY FACTOR

Recent work has demonstrated an additional cytokine known as the leukemia inhibitory factor (LIF) which may be involved in the cytokine interactions which cause the cachectic syndrome. It is also known as D-Factor, and is very similar to IL–6 in functional characteristics. (113, 114) In fact, the two cytokines both rely on the same signal transduction component, gp130, within their receptor complexes. (115) LIF has been purified from the supernatants of a number of human and animal tumor cells. (116) Like IL–6, LIF is a potent stimulus of acute phase protein synthesis by the liver. When it was purified from the supernatant of human squamous carcinoma cells it was originally described as the hepatocyte-stimulating factor. (117, 118) Later sequencing information proved this factor to be identical to LIF. Like the majority of putative cachectic mediators LIF has been proven to inhibit LPL. (119) Several *in vivo* studies support the role of LIF in cachexia. A human melanoma cell line, SEKI, constituitively produces LIF. When this cell line is implanted in nude mice, they develop marked cachectic changes. (120) Similar findings were noted when mice engrafted with a transfected cell line secreting high levels of LIF. These animals develop a fatal syndrome characterized by cachexia, excess bone formation, pancreatitis, and thymic atrophy. (121)

Another similarity to IL–6 appears to be the stimulation of LIF production by other cytokines. In our laboratory we have found that a number of murine sarcoma cell lines produce low levels of LIF on a constitutive basis. In at least one of these cell lines, nanogram quantities of TNF increase LIF production by the tumor cells by 100-fold. There is evidence that LIF and IL–6 are involved in an interactive network that develops within the tumor microenvironment (Fig. 1.2). The tumor cell appears to produce an initiating signal which leads infiltrating host inflammatory cells to produce a spectrum of cytokines particularly IL–1 and TNF. These cytokines may act locally or activated macrophages may travel to remote locations to exert cytokine effects distant from the tumor. Local cytokine production by host cells within the tumor appears to stimulate tumor cells to produce a range of secondary cytokines including IL–6 and LIF. Because production of these mediators is substantially up-regulated, they may provide the most significant mediating agents in the cachectic syndrome. Although the specific cytokine agent may not be consistent from one tumor to another, the need for interaction between tumor and functional host inflammatory cells does seem to be necessary to produce cachexia.

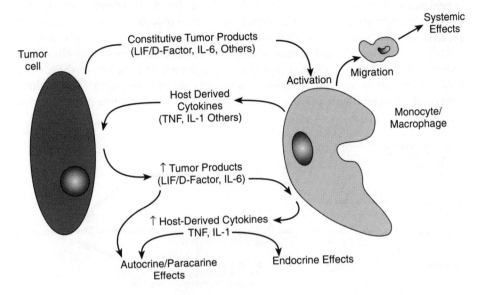

Fig. 1.2 Cytokine interactions between tumor cells and host inflammatory cells which may contribute to cancer cachexia.

MECHANISMS OF HIV-RELATED CACHEXIA

Although similar cytokine interactions appear to be at work in HIV-related cachexia, it is difficult to distinguish what effects arise from HIV infection and what is produced by the numerous infectious complications of AIDS. As indicated, TNF has been detected in the serum of AIDS patients; however no association between TNF levels and weight loss has been noted. A recent report describes a correlation between increased triglyceride levels and levels of interferon-alpha (IFN–α), but no correlation with TNF or IL–1. (122) Detailed analysis of cytokine interactions in this condition has been hampered by the lack of a small animal model of AIDS.

A component of the wasting observed in AIDS patients appears to be related to deficits in nutrient absorption. (123) In the majority of cases, malabsorption is related to intestinal infection. Protozoal organisms are the most common pathogens in HIV-related intestinal disease. These organisms tend to cause malabsorption by direct epithelial cell injury and cell loss. Villus atrophy eventually occurs which diminishes the effective absorptive surface area. Compensatory crypt hypertrophy occurs; however, it is not enough to offset widespread villus atrophy. (124) Cryptosporidia, Microsporidia, and Isospora are all protozoal agents which cause intestinal injury and malabsorption. (123) Mycobacterium avium intracellulare (MAI) infection of the intestine causes diffuse infiltration of the lamina propria and obstructs intestinal lymphatics with macrophages. This not only creates a barrier to absorption, but can cause a diffuse, exudative enteropathy. (125)

In some cases, AIDS patients suffer from malabsorption and small bowel injury without the presence of an identifiable infectious agent. This may be a result of direct cytotoxicity by the HIV virus. Although not definitive proof of this possibility, *in situ* hybridization techniques have provided evidence for viral infection of enterocytes. (126) Further evidence is provided by microscopic studies of the intestinal epithelium from patients the HIV-related wasting syndrome. One study demonstrated the presence of focal vacuolization in duodenal enterocytes. (107) Histologic staining characteristics indicated that these vacuoles are lipid laden. In these cells, lipid accumulation appears to arise as a sequela to HIV infection. These ultrastructural changes almost certainly contribute to the malabsorptive picture of this syndrome (Fig. 1.3).

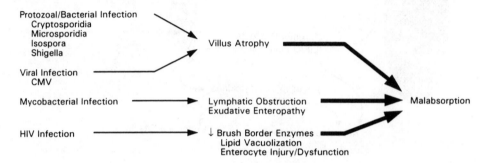

Fig. 1.3 Multiple etiologies may lead to malabsorption in AIDS patients.

In many ways the cachectic picture of HIV-related illnesses nearly parallels cancer cachexia. Many of the same cytokine mechanisms appear to be involved. However, the cytokine reactions are driven by multiple opportunistic infections and perhaps by HIV infection itself. Nutritional and digestive factors also play perhaps an even greater role than they do in cancer cachexia.

CONCLUSIONS

Despite advances in nutritional support, cancer therapy, and treatment for the infectious complications of AIDS, cachexia remains a significant problem for many patients. Early hopes that investigation would reveal a single cachectic mediator have given way to the notion that cachexia arises from a complex interaction between tumor products and multiple host-derived mediators. This interplay of signaling influences emerges clinically as progressive loss of host adipose tissue and muscle mass. We now know that there are highly specific derangements in host metabolism involving metabolic rates as well as the processing of virtually all metabolic substrates. In spite of the complexity of the interplay between tumor and host, these networks appear to rely on initiating signal cytokines which in turn lead to amplification of other cytokines or mediators. We continue to hope that if these primary signaling molecules and their receptors can be identified, they should provide the opportunity for therapeutic circumvention of many of the devastating effects of cachexia.

REFERENCES

1. DeWys WD, Begg D, Lavin PT. Prognostic effect of weight loss prior to chemotherapy in cancer patients. Am J Med 1980;69:491–9.
2. Lawson DH, Richmond A, Nixon DW, Rudman D. Metabolic approaches to cancer cachexia. Ann Rev Nutr 1982;2:277–301.
3. Nixon DW, Heymsfield SB, Cohen AE, Kutner MH. Protein calorie undernutrition in hospitalized cancer patients. Am J Med 1980;68:683–90.
4. Warren S. The immediate causes of death in the cancer. Am J Med Sci 1932;184:610–15.
5. Chlewbowski R. Significance of altered nutritional status in acquired immunodeficiency syndrome. Nutr Cancer 1985;7:85–91.
6. O'Sullivan P, Linke RA, Dalton S. Evaluation of body weight and nutritional status among AIDS patients. J Am Diet Assoc 1985;85:1483–4.
7. Kotler DP, Wong J, Pierson RN. Body composition studies in patients with the acquired immunodeficiency syndrome. Am J Clin Nutr 1985;42:1255-65.
8. Annon. What do we know about the mechanism of weight loss in AIDS? Nutr Rev 1990;48:153–5.
9. Von Roenn J, Roth E, Craig R. HIV related cachexia: potential mechanisms and treatment. Oncology 1992;49:50–4.
10. Fein R, Kelsen DP, Geller N et al. Adenocarcinoma of the esophagus and gastroesophageal junction: results of therapy and prognostic variables. Cancer 1985;56:2512–19.
11. Stovroff MC, Fraker DL, Swedenborg JA, Norton JA. Cachectin/tumor necrosis factor: a possible mediator of cancer anorexia in the rat. Cancer Res 1988;48:4567–72.
12. Darling G, Fraker DL, Jensen JC, Gorschboth CM, Norton JA. Cachectic effects of recombinant human tumor necrosis factor in rats. Cancer Res 1990;50:4008–13.
13. Balkwill F, Osborne R, Burke F et at. Evidence for tumor necrosis factor/cachectin production in cancer. Lancet 1987;2:1229–32.
14. Socher SH, Martinez D, Craig JB, Kuhn JG, Oliff A. Tumor necrosis factor not detectable in patients with clinical cancer cachexia. J Narl Cancer Inst 1988;80:595–8.
15. Moldawer LL, Lundholm CD, Lundholm K. Monocytic production and plasma bioactivities of interleukin–1 and tumor necrosis factor. Eur J Cell Biol 1988;18:486–92.
16. Splinter TA. Cachexia and cancer: a clinician's view. Ann Oncol 1992;3:S25–7.
17. Centers for Disease Control. Revision of the CDC case surveillance definition for acquired immunodeficiency syndrome. MMWR 1987;36:35–145.
18. Oliff A, Defeo-Jones D, Boyer M et al. Tumors secreting human TNF/cachectin induce cachexia in mice. Cell 1987;50:555–63.
19. Moldawer LL, Andersson C, Gelin J et al. Regulation of food intake and hepatic protein synthesis by recombinant derived cytokines. Am J Physiol 1988;254:6450–6.
20. Shamberger RC, Brennan MF, Goodgame JT, Jr, Lowry SF. A prospective, randomized study of adjuvant parenteral nutrition in the treatment of sarcomas: results of metabolic and survival studies. Surgery 1984;96:1–13.
21. DeWys WD. Anorexia as a general effect of cancer. Cancer 1979;43:2013–9.
22. Bernstein IL. Learned taste aversions in children receiving chemotherapy. Science 1978;200:1302–3.
23. Carson JA, Gormican A. Taste acuity and food attitudes of selected patients with cancer. J Am Diet Assoc 1977;70:361–5.
24. Bruera E, Catz Z, Hooper R, Lentle B. Chronic nausea and anorexia in patients with advanced cancer: a possible role for autonomic dysfunction. J Pain Symptom Manage 1987;2:19–21.
25. Cori CF, Cori GT. The carbohydrate metabolism of tumors. II. Changes in the sugar, lactic acid, and CO^2-combining power of blood passing through a tumor. J Biol Chem 1925;65:397–405.

26. Brennan MF. Uncomplicated starvation versus cancer cachexia. Cancer Res 1977;37: 2359–66.
27. Heber D, Byerly LO, Tchekmedyian NS. Hormonal and metabolic abnormalities in the malnourished cancer patient: effects on host tumor interaction. J Parent Ent Nutr 1992;16:605–45.
28. Muller JM, Brenner U, Dienst C, Picklmaier H. Preoperative parenteral feeding in patients with gastrointestinal carcinoma. Lancet 1982;1:68–71.
29. Williams RH, Heatley RV, Lewis M. Proceedings: a randomized controlled trial of pre-operative intravenous nutrition in patients with stomach cancer. Br J Surgery 1976;63:667.
30. Preshaw RM, Attisha RP, Hollingworth WJ. Randomized sequential trial of parenteral nutrition in healing of colonic anastomoses in man. Can J Surgery 1979;22:437–9.
31. Hyltander A, Drott C, Körner U, Sandstrom R, Lundholm K. Elevated energy expenditure in cancer patients with solid tumors. Eur J Cancer 1991;27:9–15.
32. Hansell DT, Davies JW, Shenkin A, Burns HJ. The oxidation of body fuel stores in cancer patients. Ann Surgery 1986;204:637–42.
33. Peacock JL, Inculet RI, Corsey R, Ford DB, Rumble WF, Lawson D, Norton JA. Resting energy expenditure and body cell mass alterations in noncachectic patients with sarcomas. Surgery 1987;102:465–72.
34. Fredrix EWHM, Soefers PB, Wonters EFM et al. Energy balance in relation to cancer cachexia. Clin Nutr 1990;9:319–24.
35. Melchoir JF, Salmon D, Rigeud P et al. Resting energy expenditure is increased in stable, malnourished HIV infected patients. Am J Clin Nutr 1991;53:437–41.
36. Homes MJT, Romjin JA, Godfried MH et al. Increased resting energy expenditure in human immunodeficiency virus infected men. Metabolism 1990;39:1186–90.
37. Holroyde CP, Gabuzda TC, Putnam RC et al. Altered glucose metabolism in metastatic carcinoma. Cancer Res 1975;35:3710–14.
38. Weinhouse S. Metabolism and isoenzyme alterations in experimental hepatomas. Fed Proc 1973; 32:2162–7.
39. Morrison SD, Moley JF, Norton JA. Contribution of inert mass to experimental cancer cachexia in rats. J Natl Cancer Inst 1984;73:991–8.
40. Eden E, Edstrom S, Bennegard K, Schersten T, Lundholm K. Glucose flux in relation to energy expenditure in malnourished patients with and without cancer during periods of fasting and feeding. Cancer Res 1984;44:1718–24.
41. Burt ME, Lowry SF, Gorschboth C, Brennan MF. Metabolic alterations in a noncachectic animal tumor system. Cancer 1981;47:2138–46.
42. Norton JA, Burt ME, Brennan MF. *In vivo* utilization of substrate by human sarcoma-bearing limbs. Cancer 1980;45:2934–9.
43. Klein S, Wolfe R. Whole body lipolysis and triglyceride-fatty acid cycling in cachectic patients with esophageal cancer. J Clin Invest 1990;86:1403–8.
44. Holroyde CP, Axelrod RS, Skutchos CC, Heff AC, Paul P, Reichard GA. Lactate metabolism in patients with colorectal cancer. Cancer Res 1979;39:4900–4.
45. Bennegard K, Eden E, Ekman L, Scherstein T, Lundholm K. Metabolic balance across the leg in weight-losing cancer patients compared to depleted patients without cancer. Cancer Res 1982;42:4293–9.
46. Albert JD, Lespagi A, Horowitz GD, Tracey KJ, Brennan MF, Lowry SF. Peripheral tissue metabolism in men with varied disease states and similar weight loss. J Surg Res, 1986;40:374–81.
47. Richtsmeier WJ, Dauchy R, Lauer AL. *In vivo* nutrient uptake by head and neck cancers. Cancer Res 1987;47:5230–3.
48. Rochester DF, Wichern WA, Fritts HW et al. Arteriovenous differences of lactate and pyruvate across healthy and diseased luman lung. Am Rev Respirat. Dis 1973;107:442–8.
49. Rhodenburg GL, Bernhard A, Krehbiel O. Sugar tolerance in cancer. JAMA 1919;72: 1528–34.

50. Glicksman AS, Rawson RW. Diabetes and altered carbohydrate metabolism in patients with cancer. Cancer 1956;9:1127–34.

51. Norton JA, Maher M, Wesley R, White D, Brennan MF. Glucose intolerance in sarcoma patients. Cancer 1984;54:3022–7.

52. Grunfeld C. Kotler DP, Hamadeh R et al. Hypertriglyceridemia in the acquired immunodeficiency syndrome. Am J Med 1989;86:27–31.

53. Shulman GI, Rothman DG, Jue T, Stein P, DeFronzo RA, Shulman RG. Quantitation of muscle glycogen sysnthesis in normal subjects and subjects with non insulin dependent diabetes by 13c neuter mycrostic resonance spectroscopy. New Engl J Med 1990; 332:223–8.

54. Lundholm K, Holm G, Schersten T. Insulin resistance in patients with cancer. Cancer 1978;38:4665–70.

55. Siddiqui RA, Williams JF. The resulation of fatty acid and branched chain amino acid oxidation in cancer cachectic rats: a proposed role for a cytokine, eicosanoid and hormone trilogy. Biochem Med Metab Biol 1989;42:71–86.

56. Eden E, Edstrom S, Bennegard K, Lindmark L, Lundholm K. Glycerol dynamics in weight-losing cancer patients. Surgery 1985;97:176–84.

57. Jeervanandam M, Horowitz A, Lowry S, Brennan MF. Cancer cachexia and the rate of whole body lipolysis in man. Metabolism 1986;35:304–10.

58. Smith KL, Tisdale MS. Increased protein degradation and decreased protein synthesis in skeletal muscle during cancer cachexia. Br J Cancer 1993;67:680–5.

59. Alexander HR, Lee JI, Chang TH, Burt ME. Amino acid and protein metabolism in tumor bearing rats. J Surg Res 1991; submitted.

60. Arbeit JM, Gorschboth CM, Brennan MF. Basal amino acid concentrations and the response to incremental glucose infusion in tumor bearing rats. Cancer Res 1985;45: 6296–6300.

61. Inculet RI, Stein RP, Peacock JL, Leskiw M, Maher M, Gorschboth CM, Norton JA. Altered leucine metabolism in noncachectic sarcoma patients. Cancer Res 1987;47: 4746–9.

62. Jeevanandam M, Horowitz GD, Lowry SF, Brennan MF. Cancer cachexia and protein metabolism. Lancet 1984;1:1423–6.

63. Fearon KCH, Borland W, Preston T et al. Cancer cachexia: influence of systemic ketosis on substrate levels and nitrogen metabolism. Am J Clin Nutr 1988;47:42.

64. Heber D, Chlewbowski TR, Ishibachi DE, Herrold JN, Block JB. Abnormalities in glucose and protein metabolism in non-cachectic lung cancer patients. Cancer Res 1982;42:4815–19.

65. Starnes HF Jr, Warren RS, Brennan MF Protein synthsis in hepatocytes isolated from patients with gastrointestinal malignancy. J Clin Invest 1987;80:1384–90.

66. Perlmutter DH, Dinarello CA, Punsel PI. Cachectin/tumor necrosis factor regulates hepatic acute gene expression. J Clin Invest 1986;78:1349–54.

67. Lundholm K, Bylund AC, Holm J, Scherston T. Skeletal muscle metabolism in patients with malignant tumor. Eur J Cancer 1976;12:465–73.

68. Jeevanandam M, Horowitz G, Lowry S, Brennan MF. Cancer cachexia and the rate of whole body lipolysis in man. Metabolism 1986;35:304–10.

69. Kotler DP, Tierney AR, Dilmonian FA et al. Correlation between total body potassium and total body nitrogen in patients with acquired immunodeficiency syndrome. Clin Res 1991;39:649A.

70. Norton JA, Moley JF, Green MV, Carson RE, Morrison SD. Parabiotic transfer of cancer anorexia/cachexia in male rats. Cancer Res 1985;45:5547–52.

71. Illig KA, Maronian N, Peacock JL. Cancer cachexia is transmissible in plasma. J Surg Res 1992;52:353–8.

72. Guy MW. Serum and tissue fluid lipids in rabbits experimentally infected with trypanosoma brucei. Trans R Soc Trop Med Hyg 1975;69:429.

73. Rouzer CA, Cerami A. Hypertriglyceridemia associated with *Trypanosoma bruceibrucei* infection in rabbits: role of defective triglyceride removal. Mol Biochem Parasitol 1980;2:31–8.

74. Kawakami BM, Cerami A. Studies of endotoxin-induced decrease in lipoprotein lipase activity. J Exp Med 1981;154:631–9.

75. Beutler B, Cerami A. Cachectin and tumor necrosis factor as two sides of the biological coin. Nature 1986;320:584–8.

76. Carswell EA, Old LJ, Kessel RJ, Green S, Fire N, Williamson B. An endotoxin induced serum factor that causes necrosis of tumors. Proc Natl Acad Sci USA 1975;72:3666–70.

77. Selby PJ, Hobbs S, Viner C, Jocieson E, Smith IE. Endogenous tumor necrosis factor in patients. Lancet 1988;1:483 (letter).

78. Lahdevirta J, Maury CPJ, Teppo AM, Repo H. Elevated levels of circulating cachectin/tumor necrosis factor in patients with acquired immune deficiency syndrome. Am J Med 1988;85:289–91.

79. Reddy MM, Sorrell SJ, Lange M, Frieco MH. Tumor necrosis factor and HIV P24 antigen in the serum of HIV-infected population. J AIDS 1988;1:436–40.

80. Grunfeld C, Kotler DP, Shigenage JK et al. Circulating alpha interferon levels and hypertriglyceridemia in the acquired immunodeficiency syndrome. Am J Med 1991;90:154–62.

81. Hommes M, Romija JA, Godfried MH et al. Increased resting energy expenditure in human immunodeficiency virus. Metabolism 1990;39:1186–90.

82. Fraker DL, Stovroff MC, Merino MJ, Norton JA. Tolerance to tumor necrosis factor in rats and the relationship to endotoxin tolerance and toxicity. J Exp Med 1988;168:95–105.

83. Socher SM, Friedman A, Martinez D. Recombinant human tumor necrosis factor induces acute reductions in food intake and body weight in mice. J Exp Med 1988;167:1957–62.

84. Tracey KJ, Morgello S, Koplin B et al. Metabolic effects of cachectin/tumor necrosis factor are modified by site of production. J Clin Invest 1990;86:2014–24.

85. Torti FM, Dieckmann B, Beutler B, Cerami A, Ringold GM. A macrophage factor inhibits adipocyte gene expression: an *in vitro* model of cachexia. Science 1985;229:867–9.

86. Feingold KR, Grunfeld C. Tumor necrosis factor-alpha stimulates lipogenesis in the rat *in vivo*. J Clin Invest 1987;80:184–90.

87. Sherman ML, Spriggs DR, Arthur KA, Imamura K, Frei E III, Kufe DW. Recombinant human tumor necrosis factor administered as a five-day continuous infusion in cancer patients: phase I toxicity and effects of lipid metabolism J Clin Oncol 1988;6:344–50.

88. Goodman MN. Tumor necrosis factor induces skeletal muscle protein breakdown in rats. Am J Physiol 1991;260:727–30.

89. Nawebi MD, Block KP, Cheeraberti MC, Buse MG. Administration of endotoxin, tumor necrosis factor, or interleukin–1 to rats activates skeletal muscle branched-chain alpha keto acid dehydrogenase. J Clin Invest 1990;85:256–63.

90. Warren RS, Donner DB, Starnes HF, Jr, Brennan MF. Modulation of endogenous hormone action by recombinant human tumor necrosis factor. Proc Natl Acad Sci USA 1989;84:8619–22.

91. Sherry BA, Gelin J, Fong Y et al. Anticachectin/tumor necrosis factor–α antibodies attenuate development of cachexia in tumor models. FASEB J 1989;3:1956–62.

92. Gelin J, Moldawer LL, Lonnroth C, Sherry B, Chizzonite R, Lundholm K. Role of endogenous tumor necrosis factor α and interleukin–1 for experimental tumor growth and the development of cancer cachexia. Cancer Res 1991;51:415–21.

93. Bendtzen K. Interleukin–1, interleukin–6 and tumor necrosis factor in infection, inflammation and immunity. Immunol Lett 1988;19:183–92.

94. Moldawer LL, Georgieff M, Lundholm K. Interleukin–1, tumor necrosis factor-alpha(cachectin) and the pathogenesis of cancer cachexia. Clin Physiol 1987;7:263–274.

95. Le J, Vilcek J. Tumor necrosis factor and interleukin–1: cytokines with multiple overlapping biological activities. Lab Invest 1987;56:234–48.

96. Dinarello CA. Biology of interleukin–1. FASEB J 1988;2:108–15.
97. Hellerstein MC, Meydani SN, Meydani M, Wu K, Dinarello CA. Interleukin–1-induced anorexia in the rat. J Clin Invest 1989;84:228–35.
98. Uehara A, Sekiya C, Takasugi Y, Namiki M, Arimura A. Anorexia induced by interleukin–1: involvement of corticotropin-releasing factor. Am J Physiol 1989;257: R613–17.
99. Lonroth C, Moldawer L, Gelin J, Kindblom L, Sherry B, Lundholm K. Tumor necrosis factor–α and interleukin 1 α production in cachectic tumor bearing mice. Int J Cancer 1990;46:889–96.
100. Tredget EE, Yu YM, Zhong S et al. Role of interleukin–1 and tumor necrosis factor in energy metabolism in rabbits. Am J Physiol 1988;255:E760–8.
101. Pomposelli JJ, Flores EA, Bistrian BR. Role of biochemical mediators in clinical nutrition and surgical metabolism. J Parent Ent Nutr 1988;12:212–18.
102. Argiles JM, Lopez-Soriano FJ, Wiggins D, Williamson DH. Comparative effects of tumor necrosis factor a (cachectin), interleukin–1–β and tumor growth on amino acid metabolism in the rat in vivo. Absorption and tissue uptake of a-amino [14C]isobutyrate. Biochem J 1989;261:357–62.
103. Warren RS, Starnes HF, Alcock N, Calvano S, Brennan MF. Hormonal and metabolic response to recombinant human tumor necrosis factor in rat: in vitro and in vivo. Am J Physiol 1988;255: E206–12.
104. Argiles JM, Lopez-Soriano FJ, Evans RD, Williamson DH. Interleukin–1 and lipid metabolism in the rat. Biochem J 1989;259:673–8.
105. Strassmann G, Masui Y, Chizzonite R, Fong M. Mechanisms of experimental cancer cachexia local involvement of IL–1 in colon 26 tumor. J Immunol 1993;150:2341–5.
106. Helfgott DC, Tatter SB, Santhanem IU et al. Multiple forms of Ifn B2/IL–6 in serum and body fluids during acute bacterial infection. J Immunol 1989;142:948–53.
107. Patterson, BU, Ehrenpreis ED, Yokoo H. Focal enterocyte vacuolization. A new microscopic finding in the acquired immune deficiency wasting syndrome. Am J Clin Pathol 1993;99:247.
108. Jablons DM, McIntosh JK, Mulé JJ. Induction of interferon–2/interleukin–6 by cytokine administration and detection of circulating interleukin–6 in the tumor bearing state. Ann NY Acad Sci 1989;557:157–60.
109. Strassmann G, Fong M, Kenney JS, Jacob CO. Evidence from the involvement of interleukin–6 in experimental cancer cachexia. J Clin Invest 1992;89:1681–4.
110. Strassmann G, Jacob C, Evans R, Beell D, Fong M. Mechanisms of experimental cancer cachexia interaction between mononuclear phagocytes and colon 26 carcinoma and its relevance to IL–6 mediated cancer cachexia. J Immunol 1992;148:3674–8.
111. Patton JS, Shepard HM, Wilking H. Interferons and tumor necrosis factor have similar catabolic effects on 3T3LI cells. Proc Natl Acad Sci USA 1986;83:8313–17.
112. Langstein HN, Doherty GM, Fraker DL, Buresh CM, Norton JA. The roles of interferon-gamma and tumor necrosis factor in an experimental rat model of cancer cachexia. Cancer Res 1991;51:2302–6.
113. Gearing DP, Thut CJ, VandenBos T et al. Leukemia inhibitory factor receptor is structurally related to the IL–6 signal transducer, gp130. EMBO J 1991;10:2839–48.
114. Hilton DJ, Gough NM. Leukemia inhibitory factor: a biological perspective. J Cell Biochem 1991;46:21–26.
115. Gearing DP, Thut CJ, Vendenbos T et al. Leukemia inhibitory factor receptor is structurally related to the IL–6 signal transducer. EMBO J 1991;10:2839–48.
116. Gascon H, Anagon I, Praloren V, Naulet J, Godard A, Soulillou SP, Jacques Y. Constitutive production of human interleukin DA cells/leukemia inhibitory factor by human tumor cell lines derived from various tissues. J Immunol 1990;7:2592–8.
117. Baumann H, Wong GG. Hepatocyte-stimulating factor III shares structural and functional identify with leukemia-inhibitory factor J Immunol 1989;143:1163–7.

118. Hilton DJ, Nicola NA, Metcalf D. Specific binding of murine leukemia inhibitory factor to normal and leukemic monocytic cells. Proc Natl Acad Sci USA 1988;85:5971–5.
119. Mori M, Yamaguchi K, Abe K. Purification of a lipoprotein lipase-inhibiting protein produced by a melanoma cell line associated with cancer cachexia. Biochem Biophys Res Commun 1989;160:1085–92.
120. Mori M, Yamaguchi K, Hondu S, Nagasuki K, Ueder M, Abe O, Abe K. Cancer cachexia syndrome developed in nude mice bearing melanoma cells producing leukemia inhibitory factor. Cancer Res 1991;51:6656–9.
121. Metcalf D, Gearing DP. Fatal syndrome in mice congrafted with cells producing high levels of the leukemia inhibitory factor. Proc Natl Acad Sci USA 1989;86:5948–2.
122. Grunfeld C, Kotler DP, Shigenaga JK et al. Circulating interferon alpha levels and hypertriglyceridemia in the acquired immunodeficiency syndrome. Am J Med 1991;90:154–62.
123. Grunfeld C, Kotler DP. Wasting in the acquired immunodeficiency syndrome. Seminars Liver Dis 1992;12:175–87.
124. Ullrich R, Zeitz M, Heise M et al. Small intestinal structure and function in patients infected with human immunodeficiency virus (HIV): evidence for HIV induced enteropathy. Ann Int Med 1989;111:15–21.
125. Roth RI, Owen RL, Keren DF, Volberding PA. Intestinal infection with mycobecterium avium in acquired immunodeficiency syndrome (AIDS): histological and clinical comparison with Whipple's disease. Dig Dis Sci 1985;30:497.
126. Fox CH, Kotler DP, Tierney AR et al. Detection of HIV–1 RNA in intestinal lamina propria of patients with AIDS and gastrointestinal disease. J Infect Dis 1989;159:467–71.

2

Chronic nausea

Jose Pereira and Eduardo Bruera

INTRODUCTION

Chronic nausea is a frequent and very distressing symptom in patients with advanced cancer. The prevalence of chronic nausea reported in the literature varies from 21 to 68%. Reuben and Mor, (1) using data from the National Hospice Study, reported nausea and vomiting in 62% of cancer patients, with a prevalence of 40% in the last 6 weeks of life. Doyle (2) found a 55% prevalence of nausea and vomiting in terminal cancer patients, while Coyle et al. (3) reported nausea in 12% of patients 4 weeks before death and in 13% 1 week before death. In another study, 14% of patients in the last 48 hours of life were found to have nausea and vomiting. (4) Ventafridda et al. (5) did not comment on the overall prevalence, but did report that 4% of patients required treatment to the point of sedation because of uncontrollable nausea and vomiting. Fainsinger et al. (6) found that although 71 out of 100 consecutive patients treated in a palliative care unit had chronic nausea, no patient required sedation because of intractable emesis. In our Palliative Care Program, chronic nausea occurs in 68% of patients with advanced cancer (Table 2.1). The differences in the prevalence and severity of nausea found by the various groups are probably due to divergent patient characteristics, differences in treatment, and different methods for the assessment of the presence and intensity of nausea.

Table 2.1 Prevalence of symptoms in 275 consecutive patients

Symptom	Prevalence (%)	95% confidence interval
Asthenia	90	81–100
Anorexia	85	78–92
Pain	76	62–85
Nausea	68	61–75
Constipation	65	40–80
Sedation–confusion	60	40–75
Dyspnea	12	8–16

Although chemotherapy-induced emesis has been evaluated extensively, chronic nausea associated with cancer has received very little attention. Most of the knowledge that exists today on the pathophysiology, emetic pathways, neuro-transmitters, and treatment modalities originate from research done on chemotherapy- and radiotherapy-induced emesis as well as post-operative nausea and vomiting.

There is no consensus on the definition of 'chronic' nausea. For the purpose of research, it is often defined as nausea existing for longer than 4 weeks. However, in a population with terminal cancer and a short life expectancy, this period may be too long. The presence of nausea for more than one week in the absence of a well-identified and self-limiting cause such as chemotherapy or radiation therapy will be used for the purpose of this review.

MECHANISMS

Chronic nausea in patients with advanced cancer is likely to be a multicausal syndrome (Table 2.2). There is increasing evidence to suggest that it may be a component of the cachexia syndrome of which the clinical manifestations include anorexia, chronic nausea, asthenia, changing body image, autonomic failure. Unfortunately, the cause is frequently difficult to determine with certainty.

Table 2.2 Frequent causes of chronic nausea in cancer

1.	Autonomic failure (gastroparesis)
2.	Opioid therapy
3.	Bowel obstruction
4.	Metabolic abnormalities (hepatic and renal failure, electolyte imbalance)
5.	Increased intracranial pressure
6.	Constipation
7.	Radiation therapy
8.	Delayed chemotherapy-induced emesis
9.	Gastric/peptic ulcer
10.	Other drugs

Autonomic failure

Patients with autonomic dysfunction frequently show symptoms ascribed to gastroparesis; mostly chronic nausea, anorexia, and early satiety. These characteristics are frequently present in advanced cancer patients. Autonomic dysfunction, as a clinical syndrome, includes cardiovascular and gastrointestinal manifestations. The cardiovascular features include postural hypotension, syncope, and a fixed heart rate. Gastrointestinal symptoms present as nausea, anorexia, constipation, or diarrhea. This syndrome was described originally in patients with neurological disorders, chronic renal disease, and diabetes mellitus. (7–9) However, isolated reports have described the presence of autonomic insufficiency in patients with advanced cancer.

Kris *et al.* (10) reported to ten cancer patients complaining of chronic nausea and vomiting and found to have delayed gastric emptying. Our group studied the incidence of cardiovascular autonomic insufficiency in 43 patients with advanced breast cancer and 20 normal sex- and age-matched controls. Autonomic failure was present in 52% of cases in the patient group, compared to 7% in the control group. Among the cancer patients, autonomic failure was more common in those with poor performance status and malnutrition. (11) In a further study which included five patients with advanced cancer complaining of unexplained chronic nausea and anorexia, 16 out of 23 tests of autonomic function were abnormal, compared with none of 25 tests performed in five healthy adult controls. (12) None of the five patients had clinical or laboratory evidence of disseminated disease to the abdomen, including the liver, and all had normal endoscopy and barium meals, suggesting no mucosal injury. All five patients had sever gastroparesis (mean emptying time 192 ± 28 minutes) as compared to five controls (mean emptying time 66 ± 5 minutes) when assessed with a gastric emptying scan. The differences between the patients and controls were statistically significant and it was concluded that gastroparesis was the cause of chronic nausea and anorexia in these patients. There have been several other cases reported in the literature of autonomic dysfunction associated with lung and pancreas cancers. (13–16)

The cause of this autonomic dysfunction remains to be established, but appears to have a multifactorial etiology. Malnutrition *per se* has been suggested as a cause of autonomic neuropathy. (7) It is interesting to note that Jewish physicians in the Warsaw Ghetto during the Second World War found that their starving patients were not able to increase their blood pressure with effort and had a constant tachycardia with no change upon standing up. (17) Features of autonomic dysfunction have also been described in patients with anorexia nervosa. Furthermore, studies on animals have suggested that fasting suppresses the activity of the sympathetic nervous system. (18)

There are isolated case reports suggesting autonomic dysfunction as a paraneo-plastic manifestation of advanced cancer. (14, 19, 20) Park *et al.* (19) reported a patient with bronchial carcinoma who showed postural hypotension and abnormal tests for autonomic dysfunction that disappeared after irradiation of the tumor. In a second report, a patient with small cell carcinoma of the lung developed intestinal pseudo-obstruction and abnormal tests for autonomic dysfunction. An autopsy demonstrated degeneration of autonomic nerves without tumor involvement in the area. Antineuronal antibodies have also been identified in patients with small cell lung carcinoma who demonstrated neurological signs consistent with autonomic neuropathy. (21)

Direct tumor involvement may also be a possible etiological factor in autonomic neuropathy. (22) Radiation damage to the autonomic ganglia may potentially also play a role. However, its contribution has not been well defined, but the amount of radiation damage to the ganglia is determined primarily by the dose fractionation schedule and volume irradiated. (23) Our group has noted cardiovascular autonomic neuropathy after the administration of chemotherapeutic agents, vinca-alkaloid being the most commonly involved. (24) Furthermore, drugs such as opioids, antidepressants, anticholinergics, and vasodilators, occasionally used in the treatment of cancer-related symptomatology, may also cause adverse effects on the autonomic system. HIV infection has also been noted to produce autonomic insufficiency. (25)

Autonomic dysfunction is, therefore, a frequent feature in advanced cancer and should be suspected mainly in patients with unexplained tachycardia, low performance status, chronic nausea, and malnutrition (Table 2.3).

Table 2.3 Possible causes of autonomic dysfunction in cancer patients

1. Malnutrition
2. Paraneoplastic phenomenon
3. Tumor invasion of nervous tissue
4. Chemotherapeutic agents, e.g. vinca-alkaloids
5. Other drugs, e.g. anticholinergics
6. Radiotherapy
7. Idiopathic

Role of opioids in chronic nausea

Opioid analgesia can cause nausea in patients after initiation or increase in dose. These patients usually present with short-lasting emesis that responds well to most anti-emetics. Short-lasting, reversible nausea may be experienced initially. Some patients, particularly those receiving high doses of opioids, experience chronic and severe nausea that may be accompanied by abdominal pain, constipation, and gas distension of the large bowel and occasionally the small bowel. (26, 27) Several possible mechanisms of opioid-associated nausea have been postulated. These include vestibular stimulation, (28, 29) delayed gastric emptying, (30) opioid-induced constipation, and direct stimulation of the chemoreceptor trigger zone. (31, 32) The chemoreceptor trigger zone is located in the area postrema and appears to have one of the highest densities of opioid receptors. (33) The presence of opioid receptors in the area postrema is consistent with the observation of morphine- and enkephalin-induced emesis in the dog after local or systemic administration, the later responses being abolished by ablation of the area postrema. (34) Morphine and related mu-agonists also have appreciable affinity for delta and kappa opioid receptors. (35) Opioid agonist stimulation of delta opioid receptors (which are not antagonized by naloxone) can cause the release of dopamine, suggesting that at least some of the emetic effects of opioids are mediated by dopaminergic neurons.

In addition to short lasting emesis, opioids can cause chronic nausea due to the accumulation of active metabolites such as morphine–6–glucuronide (M–6–G) when the opioids have been used for long periods of time. It occurs more commonly when high doses have been used but occasionally may be encountered with low doses. (36) Metabolite accumulation may be more prevalent in the setting of renal failure. M–6–G is excreted by the kidney and several studies have demonstrated that its clearance is decreased in patients with renal insufficiency. However, cancer patients can develop sever, persistent, opioid-induced nausea while receiving only small doses of morphine.

Bowel obstruction

Bowel obstruction has been reported to occur in approximately 3% of all terminally ill cancer patients. However, it was noted to be as high as 15% in our unit. This discrepancy is probably due to the admission criteria of our Palliative Care Unit which admits only patients with severe physical and psychosocial distress. (37, 38) It is often very difficult to differentiate between complete and incomplete bowel obstruction. While an acute complete bowel obstruction is very easily diagnosed, the majority of patients appear to experience a slow progression from partial to complete bowel obstruction and some patients develop intermittent obstructive symptoms. These episodes of obstruction are often accompanied by nausea and vomiting. Duodenal expansion is a strong stimulus, via sympathetic and vagal afferents, for nausea and retching.

Constipation

Severe constipation aggravates nausea. Constipation is a frequent complication of advanced cancer, the causes of which may be immobility, decreased oral intake, dehydration, autonomic failure, and opioid analgesics and other drugs. (39) Constipation can cause a number of significant symptoms, such as abdominal pain, distension, nausea and vomiting, urinary retention, and cognitive failure. Terminally ill cancer patients have many risk factors for severe constipation and, therefore, should be carefully assessed for this complication and prophylactic measures should be taken.

Pathophysiology

There are various neural pathways and neurotransmitters involved in the emetic process and a knowledge of these could lead to rational approach to anti-emetic selection. Fig 2.1 summarizes the various potential emetic pathways and neurotransmitters involved. Since several pathways and neurotransmitters are probably often involved, several anti-emetics with different antagonistic/agonistic activity may be necessary. A large amount of knowledge regarding the emetic pathways and neurotransmitters was gained from research done in chemotherapy- and radiotherapy-induced nausea and post-operative models. (40, 41) These are easy models to research in that the inception cohort usually consists of patients who are without any nausea prior to the administration of the radio- or chemotherapy. The chemo- or radiotherapy is then initiated and a predictable course in terms of nausea follows. In chronic nausea, however, there exists many other confounding factors and insults which makes research regarding the mechanism and management more intricate and difficult. In chronic nausea, there may be additional processes involved and simple extrapolation from chemotherapy and radiotherapy modules does not render a true reflection of the processes involved in chronic nausea. It is of interest that drugs such as megestrol, metoclopramide, dexamethasone, and cannabinoids, which are used in the treatment of anorexia–cachexia syndrome, are also anti-emetics. (42, 43)

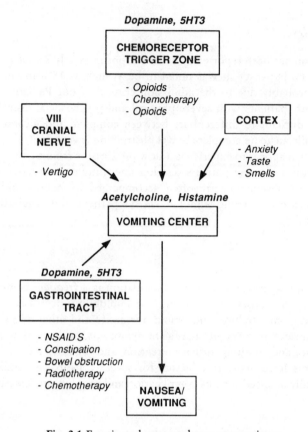

Fig. 2.1 Emetic pathways and neurotransmitters.

Nausea and vomiting are controlled by the vomiting center located in the dorsolateral reticular region of the medulla. This central, coordinating area appears to integrate various incoming signals converging from several areas and activates the emetic process. Histamine and acetylcholine appear to be the predominant neurotransmitters at this level. The areas which supply the afferent input to the emetic center are as follows:

1. The cortex and other areas such as the diencephalon and limbic system. Taste, smell, increased intracranial pressure, and psychogenic stimuli can each contribute to and evoke the vomiting response.

2. The chemoreceptor trigger zone (CTZ) is situated in the area postrema in the midbrain and it samples both blood and cerebral spinal fluid. The predominant neurotransmitters here are dopamine (D_2) and serotonin ($5-HT_3$). There is a direct link between the CTZ and the emetic center. Bacterial toxins, metabolic products (for example, uremia) and chemotherapeutic agents, and irradiation produce emesis by stimulating this zone. This, too, is the classic pathway of the apomorphine-induced vomiting mechanism. Emesis mediated by the CTZ involves dopaminergic pathways and this fact has been the basis for the major class of drugs used in the pharmacological management of nausea and vomiting;

for example, antidopaminergic drugs such as the phenothiazines, the butyro-pherones (haloperidol), and metoclopramide.

3. The upper gastrointestinal tract sends impulses to the central nervous system via vagal and sympathetic stimulation. Metastatic disease, chemotherapy drugs, irradiation, bacterial toxins, certain drugs, and gastric and duodenal expansion stimulate this route. Dopamine and acetylcholine are involved, allowing the prokinetic drugs such as metoclopramide, domperidone, and cisapride to be used. Recently 5–HT has also been found to be an important neurotransmitter at this level. The presence of serotonin neurotransmitters both in the gut and in the CTZ has resulted in the success of 5–HT_3 antagonists in the treatment of chemotherapy- or radiotherapy-induced nausea.

4. Motion stimulates the receptors of the labyrinth. Impulses are transmitted via the vestibula nucleus into the cerebellum, then to the CTZ, and then to the vomiting center. Anticholinergics and antihistamines are effective at this level since the predominant neurotransmitters are histamine and acetylcholine. Motion is seldom responsible for emesis in cancer patients.

ASSESSMENT

Nausea and vomiting are dynamic processes frequently changing in intensity. In order to achieve continuity in the management and effective follow-up the assessment should be dynamic. The assessment of chronic nausea should allow for multiple assessment and simple documentation. However, because it is a subjective symptom, the expression of its intensity will vary from patient to patient. From a practical point of view, the palliative care team will occasionally observe that the expression of nausea will not always correlate with the presumed pathophysiology of the under-lying conditions. Even though there are no 'gold standards' for nausea assessment as there are in the monitoring of hypertension (blood pressure) or diabetes mellitus (blood glucose), there are a number of highly effective assessment systems such as visual analog scales, numerical scales, and verbal descriptors. All these descriptors correlate quite well with each other. Once the intensity of nausea has been assessed, the next step is to assess it carefully within the context of other symptoms such as pain and anxiety. That is, the multidimensional aspect of the symptom has to be assessed in order to decide on the therapeutic strategy. (39) An example of such a multidimensional assessment tool is the Edmonton Symptom Assessment System (ESAS) which is based on visual analog scales looking not only at pain and nausea, but anxiety, depression, appetite, shortness of breath, and sense of well-being amongst others. (44) These tools can be used to document the intensity of the nausea, initially as a baseline assessment and then on a regular basis thereafter, giving the examiner a sense of the therapeutic effect of the management and aiding in clinical decision making. It also allows for a more reproducible assessment with intent for quality control and research.

A thorough history is mandatory and should be combined with an evaluation of clinical features and appropriate investigations in an attempt to determine the likely cause. The intensity, frequency, exacerbating and alleviating factors, and onset and duration of nausea should be documented. If there is co-existing vomiting, then the nature of the vomiting should also be reviewed. The quantity of the emesis could give a clue to the etiology. Large-volume emesis may indicate gastric outflow obstruction while small-volume emesis could indicate gastric stasis. The extent to which the emesis interferes with oral intake should be noted as large and frequent volumes of emesis put the patient at risk of rapid dehydration. Syncopal episodes and early satiety may indicate autonomic failure. Other elements in the history are important. The type of cancer which the patient has could have a bearing on the etiology of the nausea. The presence of tumors that may metastasize to the brain frequently, such as melanomas, should make one suspect raised intracranial pressure. In intra-abdominal malignancies or metastases, bowel obstruction could be suspected. The stomach and duodenum could be 'squashed' causing the squashed stomach syndrome'. Symptoms and signs of raised intracranial pressure could indicate brain metastases.

A review of drugs is imperative and the use of opioids and anticholinergics should be specifically noted. Drugs such as the non-steroidal anti-inflammatories and antibiotics may cause gastritis and mucosal damage. A history of past medical problems and present concurrent illnesses is important. Peptic ulcer disease is an example here of a concurrent medical illness which may cause nausea and vomiting. Diabetic neuropathy may result in autonomic failure.

Constipation, as already indicated, is a common complication of cancer and may aggravate nausea. The frequency of bowel movements, reference to abdominal distension, rectal fullness, oozing of stool, change in the amount of gas or stool passed recently, history of laxative use, and type and dose and date of the last bowel movement should be obtained. Unfortunately, the assessment of constipation is notoriously inadequate in cancer patients. (45, 46) A more concerted effort should be made to confirm or exclude the presence of constipation. Unfortunately, clinical impression is likely to be highly unreliable and additional aids such as a plain abdominal radiograph should be used to assist in the diagnosis of constipation. (47) The purpose of the radiograph is the assessment of the amount of stool in the colon. The colon is divided into four quadrants; the ascending, transverse, descending, and rectosigmoid segments. Each segment receives a score from 0 to 3, where $0 =$ no stool seen and $3 =$ complete stool impaction of that segment. These scores are totalled, a score of 0 being the presence of no stool and a score of 12 representing stool occupying all the lumen of the four quadrants of the colon. Studies have reported this technique as sensitive and reliable for the amount of colonic stool.

Physical examination, apart from findings related directly to the cancer itself and its complications such as cachexia, may be significant of signs of bowel obstruction or findings of raised intracranial pressure such as neurological changes and papilledema. Simple tests such as blood pressure changes on standing and an absence of heart rate variation during valsalva maneuvers may signify autonomic failure.

It is also important to exclude other causes such as renal impairment, hepatic failure, and other metabolic abnormalities such as hypercalcemia and hyponatremia. Certain laboratory investigations are, therefore, appropriate. Investigations such as CT scans of the brain may be indicated where brain metastases are suspected. Abdominal X-rays are relatively simple to perform and may reveal a lot of information. Supine X-rays may indicate the presence of stools and fecal impaction and erect or decubitus views may show fluid levels and air in the bowel typical of bowel obstruction. More sophisticated investigations such as gastric emptying scans are probably not justified on a routine basis.

MANAGEMENT

The management of chronic nausea and the process of choosing an appropriate treatment modality and anti-emetic depends on the postulated cause of the nausea. The assessment is, therefore, crucial in an attempt to find a possible etiology and to target therapy. The approach to management of chronic nausea can be seen in three stages: measures to correct the underlying cause, general measures, and symptomatic treatment (pharmacological modalities with or without surgical interventions).

Correcting the underlying cause

An attempt should first be made to correct the underlying cause. Metabolic abnormalities, where possible, need to be corrected. In situations where opioids are suspected, a change of opioids using equi-analgesic doses can be expected to improve symptoms of nausea while maintaining pain control. (48) Aggressive bowel care, including cleansing enemas and regular laxatives, should be instituted when constipation stool impaction is suspected. In some cases such as brain metastases, the cause of the nausea is irreversible but symptom control may be attempted with radiation therapy or drugs such as corticosteroids.

General measures

General measures include maintenance of good oral hygiene (poor oral hygiene may contribute to chronic nausea), creating a comfortable environment for the patient, regular baths to avoid noxious body odors, and attention to diet. Since early satiety is a common problem associated with chronic nausea, dietary considerations could include, where tolerated, smaller volume meals at more regular intervals, low fat meals, and the avoidance of spicy foods – all these being possible triggers of nausea. (49)

Pharmacological modalities

Initial pharmacological management should be focused on the prokinetic drugs to normalize upper gastrointestinal motility. Examples of these are metoclopramide, domperidone, and cisapride. The efficacy of orally administered metoclopramide in treating delayed gastric emptying in patients who do not have cancer has been established in a number of controlled clinical trials. (50) Metoclopramide has also demonstrated efficacy in reversing tumor-associated gastroparesis (10, 51) and, in uncontrolled comparisons, anorexia and nausea associated with advanced cancer. Metoclopramide demonstrates marked D_2 receptor antagonism and weak antagonism at the $5-HT_3$ receptor. In addition to its local effects in the gastrointestinal tract, metoclopramide demonstrates potent anti-emetic properties through antagonism of

D_2 receptors in the CTZ. At high doses, metoclopramide produces 5-HT$_3$ receptor blockade, which may contribute to its anti-emetic activity. However, these high doses are impractical. Bruera *et al.* (52) demonstrated that these pharmacological effects of metoclopramide provide a rational basis for its use in chronic nausea associated with advanced cancer. Unfortunately, the short elimination half-life of metoclopramide necessitates frequent administration to provide optimal relief of nausea. The short duration of action of metoclopramide in clinical trials supports the view that sustained plasma metoclopramide concentrations are required to suppress nausea and vomiting and possibly other gastrointestinal symptoms associated with advanced cancer. As a result, some patients require frequent administration or continuous infusions for optimal results. (53) Although both metoclopramide and domperidone are antidopaminergic agents, domperidone does not cross the blood–brain barrier and has, therefore, fewer extrapyramidal side-effects than metoclopramide. Domperidone's effect is primarily on gastric emptying. The phenothiazines are another group of dopamine receptor antagonists that may be effective in the treatment of nausea, but unfortunately, may produce severe sedation limiting their use. Butyrophenones, of which haloperidol is used most frequently, block dopamine at the CTZ and are effective anti-emetics. They do not increase gastrointestinal motility and are thus the drugs of choice in complete bowel obstruction. Cisapride, is a gastrointestinal prokinetic agent whose activity is considered to be due to enhancement of the physiological release of acetylcholine at the myenteric plexus. Cisapride decreases duodenal gastric reflux and also enhances intestinal propulsive activity, improving both small and large bowel transit. It may, therefore, be a helpful agent in the management of chronic nausea associated with autonomic dysfunction and gastroparesis.

Antihistamines such as cyclizine, promethazine, and dimenhydrinate exert their effects centrally on the vomiting center and peripherally on the vestibular apparatus. They are useful if a vestibular component to the nausea is suspected. This, however, is infrequent in chronic nausea.

It is not just anti-emetics and pro-motility drugs which are useful in the management of chronic nausea. Occasionally, adjuvant medications have to be added. Corticosteroids are known to have a non-specific anti-emetic effect. In addition, they can reduce edema around tumors and this may be one mechanism whereby they can decrease nausea and vomiting. This is particularly true in brain and gastrointestinal tumors (it can be useful in radiation- and chemotherapy-induced emesis). A number of controlled and uncontrolled studies have suggested that some symptoms of cancer patients, such as anorexia and asthenia, can be alleviated by corticosteroid treatment, giving patients an increased sensation of well-being. Several authors have found a significant symptomatic improvement in both appetite and strength in patients after two weeks of dexamethasone treatment, but such improvement disappeared after four weeks of treatment. (54) Octreotide, the somatostatin analog can have a role in the control of emesis associated with gastrointestinal obstruction. (55, 56) It acts by decreasing gastrointestinal secretions and increasing gastrointestinal fluid absorption.

Since 1988, our group has been using a standard therapeutic ladder for the management of chronic nausea of cancer which includes metoclopramide and dexamethasone (Fig. 2.2). Step 1 involved the use of metoclopramide and doses of 10 mg administered orally or subcutaneously every 4 hours. Supplemental doses of metoclopramide 10 mg orally or subcutaneously were allowed every hour as needed for breakthrough nausea. This first step was chosen in view of the demonstrated anti-emetic effects of metoclopramide in patients with chemotherapy-induced emesis and autonomic failure. The 4-hourly interval was chosen because of the short half-life of metoclopramide and in order to coincide with the dosing of scheduled opioid analgesics. Step 2 involved the addition of dexamethasone 10 mg orally/subcuta-neously twice daily. This step was chosen in view of the demonstrated synergistic effect of corticosteroids with metoclopramide. (57) Step 2 treatment was adminis-tered when step 1 failed to control nausea after at least 2 days of treatment (defined as a consistent complaint of nausea by the patient plus more than two extra doses of metoclopramide per day). When step 2 failed after at least 2 days, step 3 was initiated. This step involved metoclopramide given by continuous subcutaneous infusion at a daily dose of 60–120 mg plus dexamethasone at the same dose as in step 2. This step was chosen after observation of excellent response and good tolerance to continuous subcutaneous infusion of metoclopramide in refractory chronic and chemotherapy-induced emesis. (58) Occasionally, patients with severe emesis proceeded directly from step 1 to step 3. Step 4 included a number of other anti-emetics and was employed when there were contra-indications or toxicity to either metoclopramide or dexamethasone or when the previous three steps failed to control nausea. This usually involved sequential trials of haloperidol, dimenhy-drinate, and/or cisapride.

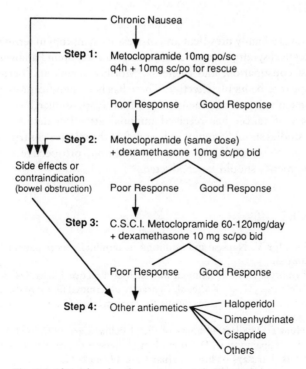

Fig. 2.2 Algorithm for the treatment of chronic nausea.

Fortunately, standard anti-emetic regimes using well-tolerated drugs such as those mentioned above, result in a high degree of success. However, sporadically, all the usually indicated anti-emetics failed. Several cases are reported in the literature of such refractory nausea responding to ondansetron, one of the new 5–HT$_3$ antagonists. (59) Although the use of ondansetron and other 5–HT$_3$ antagonists in the treatment of chemotherapy- and radiotherapy-induced nausea has been extensively researched and reported on, (60) no clinical trials are reported on the use of the 5–HT$_3$ antagonists in chronic nausea. Ondansetron's effect on serotonin-facilitated emetic pathways may lend itself to the management of chronic nausea, but further prospective clinical trials are required.

Surgical interventions

Surgical interventions may be appropriate with vomiting caused by intestinal obstruction. Procedures such as percutaneous gastrostomy for gastric outlet obstruction can greatly improve symptoms in some patients. (61, 62) Laparotomy for gastrointestinal obstruction due to tumor or adhesions can not only abolish symptoms, but improve life expectancy and quality. Surgery should be considered if a bypass procedure or excision of the obstructing lesion is possible and the patient's general condition suggests a life expectancy long enough to benefit from surgery.

CONCLUSION

Chronic nausea is a highly prevalent and distressing symptom in terminal cancer. It is likely a multicausal syndrome due to autonomic failure, opioid analgesics, metabolic abnormalities, constipation, and cachexia. Motility agents and occasionally corticosteroids appear to be highly effective. There has been significant, ongoing research in the pharmacologic management of chemotherapy-induced emesis. However, chronic nausea of cancer has received minimal attention despite its high prevalence. Future studies should attempt to best define the relative contribution of each of these factors to the overall syndrome. In addition, prospective clinical trials of different anti-emetics should be conducted.

REFERENCES

1. Reuben BD, Mor V. Nausea and vomiting in terminal cancer patients. Arch Int Med 1983;146:2021–3.
2. Doyle D. Symptom relief in terminal illness. Med Practice 1983;1:694–8.
3. Coyle N, Adelhardt J, Foley KM et al. Character of terminal illness in the advanced cancer patient: pain and other symptoms during the last 4 weeks of life. J Pain Symptom Manage 1990;5:83–93.
4. Lichter I, Hunt E. The last 48 hours of life. J Palliat Care 1990;6(4)4:7–15.
5. Ventafridda V, Ripamonti C, DeConno F et al. Symptom prevalence and control during cancer patients' last days of life. J Palliat Care 1990;6:7–11.
6. Fainsinger R, Bruera E, Miller MJ et al. Symptom control during the last week of life on a palliative care unit. J Palliat Care 1991;7(1):5–11.

7. Henrich W. Autonomic insufficiency. Arch Int Med 1982;142:339–44.
8. Ewing D, Campbell I, Clarke B. Assessment of cardiovascular effects in diabetic autonomic neuropathy and prognostic implications. Ann Int Med 1980;92:308–11.
9. Hoskins DJ, Bennett T, Hampton JR. Diabetic autonomic neuropathy. Diabetes 1978; 27:1043–54.
10. Kris M, Yeh S, Gralla RJ et al. Symptomatic gastroparesis in cancer patients. A possible cause of cancer associated with anorexia (abstract). Proc Am Soc Clin Oncol 1985;4:C–1038, 267.
11. Bruera E, Chadwick S, MacDonald N et al. Study of cardiovascular autonomic insufficiency in advanced cancer patients. Cancer Treat Rep 1986;70(12):1383–7.
12. Bruera E, Catz Z, Hooper R et al. Chronic nausea and anorexia in patients with advanced cancer: a possible role for autonomic dysfunction. J Pain Symptom Manage 1987;2(1):19–21.
13. Walsh J, Low P, Allsop J. Autonomic disturbances produced by lung cancer: a report of two unusual cases. Proc Aust Assoc Neurol 1975;12:81–3.
14. Schuffer M, Wallace H, Fleming C et al. Intestinal pseudo-obstruction as the presenting manifestation of small cell carcinoma of the lung: paraneoplastic neuropathy of the gastrointestinal tract. Ann Int Med 1983;98:129–34.
15. Thomas J, Shields R. Associated autonomic dysfunction and carcinoma of the pancreas. BMJ 1970;4:32.
16. Gould GA, Ashworth M, Lewis GT. Are cardiovascular reflexes more commonly impaired in patients with bronchial carcinoma? Thorax 1986;41:372–5.
17. Apfelbaum–Kowalski E. Pathophysiology of the circulatory system in hunger disease. In: Hunger disease: studies by the Jewish Physicians in the Warsaw Ghetto (ed. Winnick M). New York: John Wiley and Sons, 1979:125–60. (Translated from Polish by Martha Osnis.)
18. Bleich H, Boro E, Fasting, feeding and regulation of the sympathetic nervous system. New Engl J Med 1978;298:1295–1300.
19. Park D, Johnson R, Crean G. Orthostatic hypotension in bronchial carcinoma. BMJ 1972;3:510–1.
20. Mamdani MB, Walsh RL, Rubino FA et al. Autonomic dysfunction and Eaton Lambert Syndrome. J Auton Nerv Syst 1985;4:315–20.
21. Anderson E, Rosenblum EK, Gravs F et al. Auto antibodies in paraneoplastic syndromes associated with small-cell lung cancer. Neurology 1988;38:1391–8.
22. Ingham J, Bernard E. Cardiovascular autonomic insufficiency in a patient with metastatic malignancy. J Pain Symptom Manage 1995;10(2):156–60.
23. Gilbert HA, Kagan AR. Radiation damage to the nervous system, a delayed therapeutic hazard, 1st edn. New York: Raven, 1980:94–5.
24. Roca E, Bruera E, Politi P et al. Vinca alkaloids-induced cardiovascular autonomic neuropathy. Cancer Treat Rep 1985;69(2):149–51.
25. Villa A, Forest V, Confalonier F. Autonomic neuropathy and HIV infection. Lancet 1987;2:915.
26. Manara L, Bianchetti A. The central and peripheral influence of opioids on gastrointestinal propulsion. Ann Rev Pharmacol Toxicol, 1985;75:249–73.
27. Bruera E, Brenneis C, Chadwick S et al. Continuous subcutaneous infusion of narcotics using a portable disposable device in patients with advanced cancer. Cancer Treat Rep 1987;71(6):635–7.
28. Rubin A, Winston J. The role of the vestibular apparatus in the production of nausea and vomiting following the administration of morphine to man. J Clin Invest 1958;24:1261–6.
29. Riding JE. Minor complications of general anesthesia. Br J Anaesth 1975;47:91.
30. Kandeel F, Mena I, Chlebowski R. Differential effects of opioids on solid-phase gastric emptying in patients with and without cancer (abstract). Proc Am Soc Clin Oncol 1993;12:1598, 459.

31. Stewart JJ, Weisbraodt NW, Burko TF. Intestinal reverse peristalsis associated with morphine-induced vomiting. In: Opiates and endogenous opioid peptides (ed. Kosterlitz HW). Amsterdam: Elsevier, 1976:46–58.

32. Inturrisi C, Hanks G. Opioid analgesic therapy. In: Oxford textbook of palliative medicine (ed. Doyle D, Hanks G, MacDonald N). Oxford: Oxford University Press, 1993:166–82.

33. Cowan A, Doxey JC, Metcalf G. A comparison of pharmacologic effects produced by leucine-enkephalin, methionine-enkephalin, morphine and ketocyclazocine. In: Opiates and endogenous opioid peptides (ed. Kosterlitz HW). Amsterdam: Elsevier, 1976:95–103.

34. Carpenter DO, Briggs DB, Strominger N. Peptide-induced emesis in dogs. Behav Brain Res 1984;11:277–8.

35. Duggan AW, North RA. Electrophysiology of opioids. Pharmacol Rev 1983;35:219–82.

36. Hagen N, Foley K, Cerbone D et al. Chronic nausea and morphine–6–glucuronide. J Pain Symptom Manage 1991;6(3):125–8.

37. Reid DB. Palliative management of bowel obstruction. Med J Aust 1988;148:54.

38. Fainsinger RL, Spachynski K, Hanson J et al. Symptom control in terminally ill patients with malignant bowel obstruction. J Pain Symptom Manage 1994;9(1):51–3.

39. Bruera E. Patient assessment in palliative cancer care. Cancer Treat Rev, Suppl Reisengburg II (In press).

40. Hesketh P. Treatment of chemotherapy-induced emesis in the 1990's: impact of the 5HT3 receptor antagonists. Support Care Cancer 1994;2:286–92.

41. Perez EA, Gandara DR. Advances in the control of chemotherapy-induced emesis. Ann Oncol 3 Suppl 1992;3:47–50.

42. Nelson KA, Walsh D, Sheehan FA. The cancer anorexia cachexia syndrome. J Clin Oncol 1994;12:213–25.

43. Coprinzi CL. Controlled trial of megestrol acetate for the treatment of cancer, anorexia and cachexia. J Natl Cancer Inst 1990;12:1127–32.

44. Bruera E, Kuehn N, Miller MJ, Selmser P, Macmillan K. The Edmonton symptom assessment system (ESAS): a simple method for the assessment of palliative care patients. J Palliat Care 1991;7(2):6–9.

45. Portenoy RK. Constipation in the cancer patient: causes and management. Med Clin North Am 1987;71:303–11.

46. Bruera E, Suarez-Almazor M, Velasco A, Bertolino M, MacDonald SM, Hanson J. The assessment of constipation in terminal cancer patients admitted to a palliative care unit: a retrospective review. J Pain Symptom Manage 1994;9(8):515–19.

47. Starreveldt JS, Pok MA, Van Wijk HJ et al. The plain abdominal radiograph in the assessment of constipation 2 Gastroenterology 1990;28:335–8.

48. de Stoutz N, Bruera E, Suarez-Almazor M. Opioid rotation (OR) for toxicity reduction in terminal cancer patients. J Pain Symptom Manage 1995;10(5):378–84.

49. S Allan. Nausea and vomiting. In: Oxford textbook of palliative medicine (ed. Doyle D, Hanks G, MacDonald N). Oxford: Oxford University Press, 1993;4.3.1:282–90.

50. McCallum RW, Ricci DA, Rakatansky H et al. A multi-centre placebo controlled clinical trial of oral metoclopramide in diabetic gastroparesis. Diabetes Care 1983;6:463–7.

51. Shivshanker K, Bennett RW, Haynne TP. Tumor-associated gastroparesis; correction with metoclopramide. Am J Surgery 1983;145:221–5.

52. Bruera E, MacEachern T, Spachynski K et al. Comparison of the efficacy, safety and pharmacokinetics of controlled release and immediate release metoclopramide for the management of chronic nausea in patients with advanced cancer. Cancer 1994;74(12): 3204–11.

53. Bruera E, Brenneis C, MacDonald RN, Michaud M. Continuous sc infusion of metoclopramide for treatment of narcotic syndrome. Cancer Treat Rep 1987;71(11):1121–2.

54. Bruera E, Fainsinger RL. Clinical management of cachexia and anorexia. In: Oxford textbook of palliative medicine (ed. Doyle D, Hanks G, MacDonald N). London: Oxford Medical Publications, 1993:330–7.

55. Mercadante S. The role of octreotide in palliative care. J Pain Symptom Manage 1993;9(6):406–11.

56. Fainsinger RL, Pisani A, Bruera E. From the literature. Use of somatostatin analogues in terminal cancer patients. J Palliat Care 1993;9(1):56–57.

57. Bruera E, Roca E, Cedaro L, Chacon R, Estevez R. Improved control of chemotherapy-induced emesis by the addition of dexamethasone to metoclopramide in patients resistant to metoclopramide. Cancer Treat Rep, 1983;67(4):381–3.

58. Bruera E, Brenneis C, MacDonald RN, Michaud M. Continuous sc infusion of metoclopramide for treatment of narcotic bowel syndrome. Cancer Treat Rep 1987;71(11): 1121–2.

59. Cole R, Robinson F, Harvey L et al. Successful control of intractable nausea and vomiting requiring combined ondansetron and haloperidol in a patient with advanced cancer. J Pain Symptom Manage 1994;9(1):48–50.

60. Butcher M. Global experience with ondansetron and future potential. Oncology 1993;50:191–7.

61. Germio B. Home support of patients with end-stage malignant bowel obstruction using hydration and venting gastrostomy. Am J Surgery 1986;152:100–3.

62. Fainsinger RL, Spachynski K, Hanson J, Bruera E. Symptom control in terminally ill patients with malignant bowel obstruction. J Pain Symptom Manage 1994;9(1):51–3.

3

Oral complications of advanced cancer

Carla Ripamonti, Alberto Sbanotto, and Franco De Conno

INTRODUCTION

Lesions of the oral cavity have a great impact on the quality of life of patients with advanced cancer. Such lesions have a considerable morbidity and interfere a great deal with both physical and psychological function. Perhaps, most importantly, these complications impair oral nutrition with variety of consequences: malnutrition, anorexia, and cachexia.

In this chapter we discuss the most frequent complications of the oral cavity, their association with cachexia, and the possible management.

INFECTIONS

Fungal infections

Candidiasis is the most frequent fungal infection in cancer patients. (1) *Candida* species are reported to be present in the normal oral flora in 40–60% of the population. (2) Positive cultures are found in approximately 75% of the asymptomatic hospitalized population; this percentage can reach 89% if repeated cultures are obtained over a period of time. (3, 4)

In patients admitted to an oncological ward, symptomatic candidiasis appeared in up to 27% and required therapy in approximately 50% of them. (5) Oropharyngeal candidiasis can be the source of regional and systemic dissemination, particularly in granulocytopenic and immunosuppressed patients. (6)

The primary pathogen is *Candida albicans,* but other *Candida* species and other fungi, including *Aspergillus,* may be involved. The development of clinically evident oral candidiasis can depend on local and/or systemic factors. They are commonly involved in other oral infections and symptoms (Table 3.1): the role of xerostomia and drugs (for example, steroids) has to be emphasized: approximately 40% of patients receiving adrenal corticosteroid therapy and approximately 30% of those receiving antibiotics develop oropharyngeal candidiasis. (7)

Oral *Candida* infection can mainly present with two different clinical pictures: the well-known, acute pseudo-membranous form (thrush) and the chronic atrophic one. The latter is characterized by erythema and oedema usually localized to the part of the palatal mucosa in contact with dentures; this particular form of candidiasis occurs in up to 65% of very elderly individuals who wear complete maxillary dentures. It is more common in women. Angular cheilitis is often present. Other clinical pictures are less frequently seen.

Table 3.1 The main factors involved in fungal infections of oral cavity

---

1. Local factors
   Wearing dentures
   Xerostomia
   Saliva composition alterations[a]
   Oral mucosa disruption[b]
   Microbial alterations
   Reduced mechanical debridement[c]
   Previous infections
   Poor oral hygiene

2. Systemic factors
   Diabetes
   Immunosuppression
   Medical therapies (e.g. steroids)
   Nutritional status alterations

---

[a] Mainly proteins and electrolytes.
[b] Radiotherapy, chemotherapy, surgery, and cancer.
[c] Comatose patients, enterally/parenterally fed patients, trismus, etc.

In advanced cancer patients a cytologic diagnosis is not generally necessary: when indicated wet-mounted potassium hydroxide preparation or Gram stain may be preformed. Immunofluorescent techniques are less useful in these patients. (8)

Either topical or systemic treatments are available: they can be used together for more severe conditions. Nystatin suspension (100 000 U/ml, 4–6 ml every 6 hours) is the classic topical treatment of oral candidiasis. It does not show prophylactic activity and results can sometimes be disappointing. (9, 10) Its action is limited to the time of contact with the mucosal surface: due to this aspect, popsicles made of nystatin diluted with water are a soothing and effective alternative. Its association with chlorexidine reduces its activity. (11)

Clotrimazole troches (10 mg five times a day) is a good alternative: it shows good antimycotic activity, even in nystatin-resistant patients. (12, 13) It is well tolerated and less expensive than nystatin. (14) Miconazole, an imidazole derivative, is another suggested topical treatment: as lozenges (250 mg four times daily) or gel (two to four times daily) it is very effective. (15, 16) The lozenges taste may be found unpleasant. Amphotericin B lozenges can also be used for oral candidiasis, but are not as successful as clotrimazole and miconazole. (17) Intravenous amphotericin is not indicated in oral *Candida* infection due to the low concentration achieved in saliva. (18) Other topical treatments, such as 0.5–1.0% gentian violet or chlorhexidine rinsing can be used for minor infections. (19)

Among systemic treatments, ketoconazole (200 mg once daily) has been replaced by the new triazole derivatives, which cause fewer side-effects. (20, 21) Fluconazole (50–150 mg once daily) and itraconazole (100–200 mg once daily) are the main new triazole derivatives. They are well absorbed by the gastrointestinal tract, with a long half-life, allowing a once daily administration. Their spectrum of action is wide, including many different fungi. They can be used in oropharyngeal candidiasis and in systemic and deep fungal infections. (22–27) The side effects are minimal. Fluconazole can be used for oropharyngeal candidiasis at a dosage of 50 mg once daily for 7–14 days. (26) It results are possibly superior to those obtained with traditional treatments like nystatin and ketoconazole (26) and its once a day schedule makes it an attractive alternative for advanced cancer patients.

Specific treatment must be accompanied by good oral hygiene (Tables 3.2 and 3.3). When indicated, drugs such as steroids, tricyclic antidepressants, or antibiotics must be stopped or reduced.

Table 3.2 Some princples of oral hygiene

1. Check oral cavity regularly.
2. Prevent side-effects of anticancer and drug therapies.
3. Keep lips, teeth, and oral mucosa moist, clean, soft, and intact.
4. Relieve pain and maintain oral intake.
5. Teach patient and relatives about good oral hygiene.

Table 3.3 Oral hygiene

PAIN

Systemic analgesics drugs – analgesic gargles with:
Benzydamine hydrochloride 0.15%, 15 ml every 2 hours
Xylocaine viscous 2%, 5–15 ml every 4 hours
Xylocaine spray 10%, every 4 hours
Aluminium hydroxide and lignocaine 2% in equal parts
Dyclomine hyrochloride
Benzocaine 20% solution
Avoid alcohol- and lemon-containing mouthwashes

HAEMORRHAGE

Treat the basic cause:
Avoid using toothbrush and dental floss.

Use a low-pressure dental jet and/or a gauze pad wrapped around a finger or a
   disposable sponge moistened in a mild solution of baking soda and water.

Gargles with
   saline solution   povidone-iodine 1%
   hexetidine 0.1%   bicarbonate of soda
   sodium perborate   cetylpyridinium
   chlorhexidine gluconate 0.2%
   H_2O_2 3–6% in water 1:4
Gargle or used soaked gauzes with antihaemorrhage drugs
   thrombine 1–2 g/day
   tranexamic acid 2–4 g/day

Bacterial infections

Few data are available concerning bacterial infections in advanced or terminal cancer patients. (28) Previous periodontal disease is frequently linked in cancer patients to bacterial oral infections. Periodontal disease is very common in the healthy population: approximately 70–80% of adults are affected by minor periodontitis. Studies in patients with acute leukaemia suggest that periodontal disease may be an important cause of death during myelosuppression. (29–31) While the common oral flora is characterized by a prevalence of Gram-positive bacteria, xerostomia, chemotherapy, radiotherapy, and immunodepression cause a shift of oral flora towards Gram-negative colonization. (32) The presence of such heterogeneous flora, including *Candida* and other species, makes bacterial cultures difficult to interpret. Small haemorrhages, pain localized to the peridontium, and fever can be present, in particular during chemotherapy. Nearby structures secondary infection can be present (30, 31) and radiographic signs of periapical abscess may exist.

The treatment of bacterial infections depends first on adequate hygiene (Tables 3.2 and 3.3). (33–35) Periodontal probing and scaling could possibly reduce post-chemotherapy oral complications: the exact role of these treatments in advanced cancer patients has to be evaluated. In acute periodontal infection, broad-spectrum antibiotics therapy is usually initiated, followed by a more precise therapy based on the bacterial cultures, if possible and indicated. Teeth debridement with 3% hydrogen peroxide and frequent rinsing are helpful. In a palliative setting the pain treatment, usually conducted by common nonsteroidal antiinflammatory drugs (NSAIDs) and topical treatments, plays a major role.

Viral infections

Herpes simplex virus (HSV), cytomegalovirus, zoster varicella virus, and Epstein–Barr virus produce the main oral viral infection. (36) The HSV is the most common: its reported incidence in patients receiving chemotherapy is the range of approximately 11 to 65%. (37–39) HSV oral lesions appear to represent recurrent and not primary infection.

Herpetic infections, particularly HSV, are manifested by the presence of yellowish lesions, easily removed from the mucosa and extremely painful, vesicles can also appear on the lips (cold sores), and fever, anorexia, and malaise co-exist. In severe infections, the pain can be so intense as to provoke complete dysphagia. The diagnosis of HSV infection is mainly clinical: some difficulties can arise from the presence of other oral affections. When indeed, exfoliative cytology permits an accurate diagnosis (95%) in a short time. (40) They should be differentiated from aphthous ulcers: a history of vesicles preceding ulcers, a location on hard gingiva and hard palate, and crops of lesions are indicated of herpetic infection, rather than aphthous ulcers.

Specific treatment of the herpes infection is provided by acyclovir. It can be administered intravenously, with few side-effects. Patients have to be hydrated and creatinine clearance monitored. (37, 41–43) Venous extravasation has to be avoided. In haematological patients lymphocytes (count >600 per mm3) and monocytes (count >250 per mm3) recovery have been shown necessary for infection to resolve. (44) In advanced cancer patients, oral and topical routes (5% acyclovir ointment) are better employed. Control of associated infections and oral hygiene are necessary (Tables 3.2 and 3.3). Chlorhexidine 0.12% twice daily rinsing may be beneficial for HSV–1 infection. (46) Extra-oral lesions may become secondarily infected: topical antibiotics are indicated.

NEUTROPENIC ULCERS

Severe neutropenia (neutrophil count < 100 mm3) is very often complicated by mouth ulcers: (46) up to 50% of patients admitted to hospital for acute leukaemia suffer from this complication. (47) The epidemiology of neutropenic ulcers in patients with advanced solid tumors in unknown. In only approximately one-third of cases can neutropenic ulcers be traced to some local factors such as drug toxicity, HSV infection, leukaemia infiltration, trauma, or haemorrhages; the remainder have no identifiable cause. (46, 47)

Ulcers appear as one or more lesions, characterized by few signs of inflammation, regular margins, and a yellowish appearance and they are not easy to remove. (46, 47) Recovery of the neutrophil count is essential for healing. (29) Topical measures for symptomatic and oral hygiene are necessary (Tables 3.2 and 3.3). Concurrent oral infections must be prevented or treated specifically.

DRUG AND RADIOTHERAPY-INDUCED STOMATITIS

The epidemiology of these conditions is complicated by the scarcity of data; moreover several pathogenetic factors may co-exist. (28, 37, 38)

Drug-induced stomatitis

Mucositis induced by chemotherapy is a common side-effect of cancer treatment: approximately 40% of patients receiving chemotherapy develop an oral problem related to treatment. (48) Patients with haematologic malignancies develop oral problems at two or three times the rate of patients with solid tumors. (48) Patients in poor oral health have a higher risk of post-chemotherapy oral infections. (49, 50)

Stomatotoxicity generally results from the non-specific inhibitory effect of the chemotherapeutic agents on mitoses of the rapidly dividing cells of the oral epithelium (direct toxicity'). It occurs approximately 5–7 days after drug adminis-tration, often a few days before the patient's haematologic nadir. Thus, the mucosal disruption provides a portal of entry for microorganisms, at the time of maximum myelosuppression and may be accompanied by haemorrhages. A wide variety of agents may product direct toxicity, notable examples including 5-Fluorouracil (5-FU), methotrexate and doxorubicin. (48) In general, mucositis is dose-related: divided doses, rather than a bolus, can reduce this problem.

Specific treatment of the oral lesions induced by chemotherapy is almost non-existent: (28) early pilot studies suggested than an allopurinol mouthwash could be an effective antidote to 5–FU-induced mucositis; a controlled study did not confirm this hypothesis. (51–53) Due to the very short serum half-life of 5–FU, mouth cryotherapy around the time of intravenous 5–FU bolus administration has been proposed.

Secondary infection prevention, oral hygiene (Tables 3.2 and 3.3), and supportive therapy are most important. Spontaneous gingival bleeding appears when platelets count falls below 10 000 cells/mm3: a topical thrombin-soaked gauze held under pressure or microcrystalline collagen may be helpful. When local measures fail, a platelets transfusion has to be evaluated: in advanced patients its role seems to be very limited.

Radiotherapy-induced stomatitis

Virtually all patients who receive radiation therapy to the head and neck develop oral side-effects of their treatment. Radiation-induced oral mucositis is characterized by xerostomia, taste alterations, diffuse erythema, pseudo-membrane formation, and ulceration. (54) Usually, a 2-week interval between initiation of therapy and stomatitis onset is needed (due to the 2 weeks renewal rate of oral mucosa). Patients may start presenting oral soreness as little as 1000 cGy into treatment. Approximately 2000 cGy are usually necessary to develop diffuse erythema. Mucositis can be very painful and can strongly reduce oral intake. However, it is self-limiting: approximately 2–3 weeks after the end of radiation treatment are necessary for healing.

Palliative treatment of mucositis

Minimizing mucosal trauma and controlling oral pain, are the main principles of a palliative treatment of mucositis. The therapeutic schedules currently used are mainly empirical and no controlled clinical studies are available. (55)

Ice chips or popsicles are soothing. Anaesthetic rinses (xylocaine viscous, benadryl, and kaopectate) may allow simple oral intake; analgesic treatment is usually necessary. Hydrogen peroxide rinsing appears helpful in removing debris and mucus from the teeth. (43) Spicy or acidic food should be avoided and soft, low-salt foods should be given. (56) Oral hygiene should be stressed: mouth care protocols, including toothbrushing, flossing, mouth rinsing, and fluoride applications, can significantly drop the frequency of oral complications (Tables 3.2 and 3.3). (57, 58) Concurrent oral infections should be strongly treated, in particular candidiasis.

Severe oral pain may require systemically administered medications. Morphine or methadone can be administered orally or parenterally. (59) In bone marrow-transplanted patients, where severe mucositis is often present, intravenous continuous morphine is routinely used by some groups, with good results. (60)

XEROSTOMIA

Xerostomia is the subjective feeling of mouth dryness not always accompanied by a detectable decrease in salivation flow. (61, 62) Few data are available on the frequency of xerostomia in patients with advanced cancer. This symptom is referred to as 'a lot' and 'awful' in 30% of the patients at the beginning of a palliative care programme. (63) It was a specific complaint in 40% of the patients at the time of admission to a hospice, but probably 100% of the patients suffer from a dry mouth at some point during the terminal stage of the disease. (64) The causes of xerostomia are enumerated in Table 3.4.

Table 3.4 Causes of xerostomia

---

1. Reduced salivary secretion caused by

   radiotherapy in the head and neck regions
   surgery in the buccal and submandibular regions
   drugs
   obstruction, infection, aplasia, and malignant destruction of salivary glands
   encephalitiis, brain tumours, neurosurgical operations, and autonomic pathways
   destruction
   hypothyroidism
   autoimmune diseases
   sarcoidosis

2. Widespread erosion of buccal mucosa caused by

   cancer
   chemotherapy, radiotherapy, and immunodeficiency
   stomatitis
   viral, bacterial, and fungal oral infections

3. Dehydration caused by

anorexia	vomiting
diarrhea	polyuria
fever	haemorrhage
O$_2$ therapy	diabetes insipidus
breathing by mouth	difficulty in swallowing
large bedsores and/or ulcers	

4. Decreased mastication

5. Depression and anxiety

A variety of symptoms may be associated with the feeling of oral dryness. In the study by Sreebny and Valdini (62) the symptoms most frequently present in 48% or more of the xerostomic subjects were the need to do something to keep the mouth moist, the need to get out of bed at night to drink water, and difficulty with speech. In 13–30% of the patients with a dry mouth it was noted that there was an association with having to keep fluids at the bedside, loss in taste acuity, difficulty with chewing dry foods, burning and tingling sensations on the tongue, the presence of cracks or fissures at the corners of the lips, and difficulty in swallowing. Most of these symptoms can cause anorexia, loss of weight, and cachexia. Patients with a dental prosthesis may find poor tolerance to them due to frequent traumatic lesions; this also produces difficulty in mastication which leads to a reduced intake of food. (65)

Saliva is a major protector of the tissues and organs of the mouth. In its absence both the hard and soft tissues of the oral cavity may be severely damaged with an increase in ulcerations, infections like candidiasis, (66) and dental decay. (67, 68) However, numerous factors, in addition to saliva, are important in oral mucosal preservation. (69) Recently, the presence of magainins, intrinsic protective components in frog skin, was described. According to Zasloff, (70) similar substances may have a protective role for mammalian mucosa. The volume of salivary fluid output is not the only factor in maintaining oral mucosal health. Differences in salivary composition in various states of health and disease have to be investigated.

Patients treated with radiotherapy for oral or head and neck cancer suffer from xerostomia from the beginning of treatment. Radiation directed at such areas can involve one or both parotid glands or the submandibular salivary glands, resulting in a marked diminution in the normal salivary flow. (71–77) This is a consequence of radiation-induced inflammation and degeneration of the acini and ducts, (72, 78) connective tissue, (79) and vascular components of the salivary glands. The most important factor affecting the post-irradiation salivary flow after a curative dose of radiotherapy seems to be the volume of the major salivary glands irradiated, (71) with that of the parotid gland being extremely important due to its higher radiosensitivity among major salivary glands. (80–82) A sharp decrease in the salivary flow usually occurs after the first week of radiotherapy treatment with a dose of approximately 10 Gy. (77, 81, 83) This decrease in the flow rate continues throughout the treatment, resulting in almost total xerostomia. (77, 81) The symptom usually persists. While one study noted a partial return of the salivary flow 8 months after the end of the radiotherapy, (76) others found minimal, if any, improvement, some years after radiotherapy. (84, 85)

After irradiation of the salivary glands, saliva becomes more viscous, (73, 78, 86, 87) undergoes a reduction in pH, (78, 88) and loses organic and inorganic components. (88, 89) The aqueous component of whole saliva is much more sharply depressed than the proteic component during the production of xerostomia. These changes compromise the lubricating protective function of saliva, reducing its capacity to act as a barrier against irritating substances or remove bacterial and cellular debris. The amount of bicarbonates also diminishes, (73, 78, 86) which further impairs the cleaning action of saliva. It is possible to observe an increase in the salivary content of Na^+, Cl^-, Mg^{2+}, and protein. (73, 78, 82)

The reduction in the salivary flow rate, (78, 90) together with these qualitative changes, can alter the oral microbial flora and result in increased growth of streptococcus, lactobacillus, and *Candida* organism. These often irreversible alterations can rapidly damage dental structures and increase tooth decay. (74, 78) In patients undergoing radiotherapy, the tooth-decaying process can be rapid and lesions can be manifest within 3–6 months. (73) The process of decay may also provoke pain in the oral cavity, thereby adding to the suffering of the patient. Loss of already decaying teeth causes further difficulty in mastication, which, added to xerostomia, may cause difficulty in swallowing and digestion. Saving the minor oral glands may play an important role in protection against new colonization by microorganisms, (82, 86, 91, 92) or against tooth decay. (93, 94)

In addition to the flow rate measurements, amylase seems to be the best indicator of salivary gland function during radiotherapy whereas albumin and lactoferrin are good indicators of inflammatory reactions often related to irradiation. (86)

A large number of drugs with xerostomic side-effects are known including antipsychotics and tricyclic antidepressants, antihistamines, anticholinergic drugs, anticonvulsants, antipsychotics, hypnotics, beta-blockers, and diuretics. (86, 95–99) Drugs may directly or indirectly reduce the flow of saliva and initiate the feeling of oral dryness. Some of these drugs induce xerostomia through parasympatholytic effects. In the study of Sreebny *et al.* (98) almost 60% of those patients with a dry mouth took xerogenic drugs.

The intake of xerostomia-inducing medications is positively correlated with age and with the total number of drugs taken daily (97, 98) and it is highest among institutionalized patients. (97) Reductions in salivation among elderly people may be related to drug use rather than to age.

Xerostomia is not generally recognized as a side-effect of morphine, (100) but clinical experience suggests that it is a common complaint of cancer patients treated with morphine. (100–103)

Xerostomia after radiation therapy may be the most difficult to treat because of the irreversible damage to the salivary glands that may occur. Current therapy for chronic xerostomia includes salivary substitutes or salivary stimulants. Water, glycerin preparations, and artificial saliva are used as substitutes for saliva, while sialogogues, sugarless candies and chewing gum are used for saliva stimulation. (104)

A lot of commercial products are available which patients use primarily as a gargle to relieve the symptoms of xerostomia but they often do not provide improvement in these symptoms. Only a small number of controlled clinical studies are available in the literature about the treatment.

Specific and palliative therapies for xerostomia are listed in Table 3.5.

LOCAL COMPLICATIONS OF ORAL TUMORS

Some local complications of cancer can greatly affect food intake and general condition.

Facial trismus

Facial trismus is the consequence of tumor invasion of masticatory muscles, usually the pterygoid. It is common in retromolar trigone lesions, in very advanced anterior tonsillar pillar and tonsillar fossa tumors, and in soft palate lesions. (105) It is often accompanied by local pain or by pain perceived in the external ear, in the pre-auricular, or in the temporal area. Occasionally, cranial nerve involvement can be present. Radiotherapy, when possible, obtains good results alleviating facial trismus and chemotherapy too can be helpful. (105) Systemic analgesics, muscle relaxants (for example diazepam), and local anaesthetic infiltration, many help when trismus depends on a painful stimulus. Oral hygiene presents many problems due to reduced access to the oral cavity (Tables 3.2 and 3.3). Cotton swabs soaked with antiseptics, sprays, and dental jet can help. Liquid or semi-solid feeding is not always possible: whenever indicated a nasogastric or a gastrostomy line could be inserted.

Table 3.5 Treatment of xerostomia

Specific treatment

 A 2% citric acid solution (Saliram) (61)
 75–100 mg nicotinic acid more than once per day (64)
 Dehydroergotamine (106)
 Pilocarpine (107–110)
 Antholetrithione ANTT (Sulfarlem) (111)
 ANTT plus pilocarpine (79)

Xerostomia caused by drugs

 Reduce the dosage and/or change the drug if possible
 Application of fluoride gel to avoid dental damage

Xerostomia caused by systemic dehydration

 Correct the cause
 Increase the liquid intake by mouth
 Hypodermoclysis (not end-stage patients)
 Make use of the IV hydration in selected patients

Palliative treatment

 Frequent oral hygiene
 Humidified air
 Suck ice cubes, vitamin C tablets, and frozen tonic water (64)
 Chew sugarless chewing gum, lemon sugar candy, acid substances, and pieces of
 pineapple (64)
 Artificial saliva
 Glycerin, cologel, and normal saline (1:1:8)
 Carboxymethyl-cellulose, sorbitol, water, sodium fluoride, menthol, minerals, and
 chlorhexidine
 Methylcellulose plus lemon essence plus water (64)
 Hydrophilic chewing gum which releases artificial saliva with a remineralizing effect
 (112)
 Mucin-containing based on bovine salivary gland extract (113)
 Dentures which include a reservoir for the release of artificial saliva (114)

Abscesses and fistulas

Infections are very common in head and neck cancer patients. They are reported to contribute to 44–46% of causes of death in this population. (115) Cellulitis, tumor infections, and orocutaneous fistula contribute approximately 22% of febrile episodes in head and neck cancers. (115) This group of patients is very often malnourished, with a previous history of alcoholism and of chronic lung disease and with decreased salivary flow and secretory IgA levels. (48) Moreover surgery, radiotherapy, and chemotherapy often seriously damage head and neck structures of these patients.

 Gram-negative shifting of oral flora, including aerobic Enterobacteriaceae and *Pseudomonas aeruginose*, is particularly important. Anaerobic Gram-negative bacteria also play an important role in head and neck infection. (116) All these aspects have to be considered when approaching the management of abscesses and orocutaneous fistulas. A simple povidone–iodine solution can be sufficient as a preventive measure in patients at risk of developing secondary bacterial infections. The same antiseptics can be used as oral medication when abscess is already present (Tables 3.2 and 3.3). In the presence of signs of sepsis or of local pain or discharge, wide-spectrum antibiotics, including metronidazole, should be administered. (116) Patient's relatives have to be carefully instructed about medication and possible emergencies (for example, massive haemorrhages).

Tumoral discharge

Many oral cavity tumors discharge causing problems in swallowing and dysphagia and create a chronic bad taste in the mouth. In some cases, radiotherapy can help this symptom, reducing the tumour mass and its secretions. If not possible, local measures have to be applied. Frequent rinsings with hydrogen peroxide can help in removing tumor debris. Benzydamine hydrochloride rinse can reduce oral cavity colonization and help patient's mouths feel cleaner. (117) Prevention and treatment of other oral problems (for example, candidiasis) is very important (Tables 3.2 and 3.3).

TASTE ALTERATION

Taste alteration comprises a reduction in taste sensitivity (hypogeusia), an absence of taste sensation (ageusia), or a distortion of normal taste (dysgeusia). The incidence of these symptoms is unknown. According to Twycross and Lack (118) between a quarter and a half of cancer patients have a diminished taste sensation. Our clinical experience suggests that taste alterations are hardly ever reported spontaneously by the patients, but many will report it as a reason for loss of appetite if specifically questioned. Patients typically report that the food is 'tasteless' or the food is 'bitter'.

Taste is mediate through organs known as taste buds, which contain approximately 50 cells and are continuously renewed. The number of taste buds decreases with age. Buds are found on the tongue, soft palate, pharynx, larynx, epiglottis and uvula, lips and cheeks, and in the upper third of the oesophagus.

The cells of the taste buds are provided with microvilli in direct communication with the oral cavity through an apical pore. A protein (gate-keeper) regulates the quantity of stimuli that pass through the pore per unit of time. Changes in the protein molecules are controlled by the equilibrium of metals and, consequently, a deficiency of some metals and in particular of zinc is associated with hypogeusia and anorexia. (119–121)

Taste information is sent by way of the fifth, seventh, ninth, and tenth cranial nerves to the medulla (nucleus of the solitary tract) and from there through the pons and thalamus to the cortical area subserving taste. Information in this pathway is also projected to the lateral hypothalamus. A lesion in any one of these areas can alter taste perception. (122) The effect of cancer on taste is unknown. The potential causes of taste alteration are listed in Table 3.6.

Taste abnormalities in cancer patients may be correlated with the site or extent of the tumor, independent of the histological type. A positive correlation exists between weight loss and the presence of an abnormal taste sensation. (123)

Disturbances in taste can also alter digestion because stimulation of the taste organs can increase salivary and pancreatic flow, gastric contractions, and bowel motility. (122) Williams and Cohen demonstrated elevated thresholds for recognition of sour (HCl), but not bitter (urea), sweet (sucrose), or salt (NaCl) tastes, in a group of patients with lung cancer, who were tested prior to chemotherapy or radiotherapy. (124) An elevated threshold of detection for all four basic tastes was reported in a group of patients with laryngeal cancer who had been examined before laryngectomy. (125)

Table 3.6 Causes of taste alteration

Local disease of the mouth and tongue caused by cancer

Partial glossectomy

Tobacco usage

Elimination of the olfactory component of the taste or cerebral lesions

Surgical removal of the palate

Damage to the nervous structures following surgery or cerebral lesions

alteration of the cell renewing or cell regenerating cycle

malnutrition	metabolic disturbances
radiotherapy	xerostomia
drugs	stomatitis and oral infections
endocrine factors (thyroidectomy, hypophysectomy, and adrenalectomy)	

Modification in the receptor cells due to alteration of saliva by metabolic agents, drugs, and radiation

Dental pathology

Bad dental hygiene

Taste alterations have been reported as a consequence of radiotherapy for tumors in the head and neck regions. The mechanism for this effect may be due to damage to the microvilli of the taste cells or to reduced salivation. Taste loss was not observed until radiation doses of 2000 cGy had been reached. (126, 127) Between 2000 and 4000 cGy, taste loss increased rapidly and at the 6000 cGy dose level over 90% relative taste loss was observed. (126) In most instances, taste acuity is partially restored 20–60 days after radiotherapy and is fully restored with 2–4 months post-radiotherapy.

Three weeks after initiation of radiotherapy, the bitter and salt qualities showed the earliest and greatest impairment and the sweet quality the least. (128)

Drugs administered to cancer patients may also alter the taste. Approximately 80 different drugs are considered responsible for taste alterations, (129) but many of these have been reported as a cause only once.

Zinc deficiency has been noted as a potential cause of anorexia, dysgeusia, or hypogeusia. Plasma zinc levels have been found to be reduced in patients with bronchial carcinoma compared to the healthy population, and zinc in leukemic cells appears to be lower than normal white blood cells. (130)

The administration of zinc has been reported to correct abnormalities of taste in some cases. (128) Copper and nickel have also been used with good results in clinical trials. No patients treated prophylactically with 25 mg of oral zinc four times a day prior to radiotherapy developed as severe a hypogeusia as those who were not treated. (131–133)

Patients suffering from taste alterations need a correct oral hygiene, a treatment to increase salivation, and suspension of the drugs that can induce or increase the symptom (Tables 3.2 and 3.3). Patients can usually take hot food with a strong smell, adding lemon or vinegar, if stomatitis or mouth ulcers are not present.

FUTURE RESEARCH

Oral cavity problems still remain a poorly investigated area in oncological and palliative care settings. We believe that many aspects of oral care need to be better defined. Some important areas of future research could be as follows.

1. The epidemiology of oral complications and their impact on the quality of life.

2. The development of standard criteria for the assessment and classification of oral cavity pathologies.

3. The long-term oral side-effects of anticancer therapies and their optimal planning (for example, radiotherapy-fractioned schedules and different kinds of ear, nose and throat (ENT) oncological surgery).

4. The interactions between oral cavity problems and anorexia, cachexia, and malnutrition.

5. The development of adequate educational tools to involve the family in the oral care of the relative.

6. The development of new specific treatments for oral cavity problems.

CONCLUSIONS AND CLINICAL GUIDELINES

Although there are no controlled clinical data supporting a close, direct relation between oral cavity complications of advanced cancer and the anorexia–cachexia syndrome, from our practice it is evident that such a relationship exists.

Infections of the oral cavity are among the most frequent complications in patients with advanced cancer. In particular oropharyngeal candidiasis is the most frequent problem, due to both the impact of anticancer therapies (steroids, radiotherapy, and chemotherapy) and the concomitant immunodepression. Specific antifungal therapy usually gives good symptom control.

Stomatitis and xerostomia, mainly due to radiotherapy and chemotherapy, are important complications of cancer therapy. Their treatment still remains a matter of palliative and supportive care and results reported by the patients are often unsatisfactory.

Taste alterations (hypogeusia, ageusia, and dysgeusia), usually reported by patients as 'tasteless food' and 'bitter food', have to be investigated by the physician every time food aversion and/or anorexia are present. The importance of this complication, usually multifactorial, is still underestimated and, apart from oral infections and metabolic disturbances, their treatment is solely a palliative one.

Complications due to the direct tumor involvement of the oral cavity (facial trismus, abscesses, and fistulas), do not allow oral food intake; the decision to perform invasive techniques for food administration (such as nasogastric tube or percutaneous gastrostomy), always requires careful attention to both survival and quality of life of the patient.

A strong effort has to be made to apply, diffuse, and implement oral hygiene principles in cancer patients. Good and regular oral hygiene appears to be very promising, possibly cheap, and maintains a patient's dignity.

REFERENCES

1. Bodey GP. Candidiasis in cancer patients. Am J Med 1984;77D:13–19.
2. Epstein JB, Truelove EL, Izutzu KT. Oral candidiasis: pathogenesis and host defense. Rev Infect Dis 1984;6:96–106.
3. Baines MJ. Control of other symptoms. In: The management of terminal disease, 2nd edn. (ed. Saunders C). London: Edward Arnold, 1984.
4. Finlay IG. Oral symptoms and *Candida* in the terminally ill. BMJ 1986;293(3):592–3.
5. Yeo E, Alvarado T, Fainstein V, Bodey GP. Prophylaxis of oropharingeal candidiasis with clotrimazole. J Clin Oncol 1985;3(12):1668–71.
6. De Gregorio MW, Lee WMF, Linker CA et al. Fungal infections in patients with acute leukemia. Am J Med 1984;73:543–8.
7. Bodey GP, Samonis G, Rolston K. Prophylaxis of candidiasis in cancer patients. Seminars Oncol 1990;17(3):24–8.
8. Lynch DP, Gibson DK. The use of Calcofluor white in the histopathologic diagnosis of oral candidiasis. Oral Surgery Oral Med Oral Pathol 1987;63:698–703.
9. Barret AP. Evaluation of nystatin in prevention and elimination of oropharingeal *Candida* in immunosuppressed patients. Oral Surgery 1984:58:148–51.
10. DeGregorio MW, Lee MW, Ries CA. *Candida* infections in patients with acute leukemia: ineffectiviness of nystatin prophylaxis and relationship between oropharyngeal and systemic candidiasis. Cancer 1982;50:2780–4.
11. Barkvoll P, Attramadal A. Effect of nystatin and chlorexidine digluconate on *Candida albicans*. Oral Surgery Oral Med Oral Pathol 1989;67:279–81.
12. Kirkpatrick CH, Alling DW. Treatment of chronic oral candidiasis with clotrimazole troches: a controlled clinical trial. New Engl J Med 1978;299:1201–3.
13. Yeo BS, Bodey GP. Oropharyngeal candidiasis treated with a troche form of clotrimazole. Arch Int Med 1979;139:656–7.
14. Quintiliani R, Owens NJ, Quercia RA et al. Treatment and prevention of oropharyngeal candidiasis. Am J Med 1984;10:44–8.
15. Roed-Petersen B. Miconazole in the treatment of oral candidiasis. Int J Oral Surgery 1978;7:558-63.
16. Brincker H. Treatment of oral candidiasis in debilitated patients with miconazole — a new potent antifungal drug. Scand J Infect Dis 1976;8:117–20.
17. de Vries-Hospers GH, van der Waaij D. Salivary concentrations of amphotericin B following its use as an oral lozenges. Infection 1980;8:63–5.
18. Holbrook WP. Sensitivity of *Candida albicans* from patients with chronic oral candidiasis. Postgrad Med J 1979;55:692–4.
19. Holmberg K. Oral mycoses and antifungal agents. Am Dentistry J 1980;4:53–61.

20. Symoens J, Moens M, Dom J et al. An evaluation of two years of clinical experience with ketoconazole. Rev Infect Dis. 1980;2:674–82.
21. Hughes WT, Bartley DL, Patterson GG, Tufenkeji H. Ketoconazole and candidiasis: a controlled study. J Infect Dis 1983;147:1060–3.
22. Saag MS, Dismukes WE. Azole antifungal agents: emphasis on new triazoles. Antimicrobial Agents Chemother 1988;32:1–8.
23. Heykants J, Michiels M, Meuldermans W et al. The pharmacokinetics of itraconazole in animals and man: an overview. In: Recent trends in the discovery, development and evaluation of antifungal agents (ed. Fromtling RA). Barcelona: JR Prou Science Publ, 1987:223–4.
24. Cauwenbergh G, DeDoncker P, Stoops K et al. Itraconazole in the treatment of human mycoses: review of three years of clinical experience. Rev Infect Dis 1987;9:S146–52.
25. Humphrey MJ, Jevenson S, Tarbit MH. Pharmacokinetic evaluation of UK-49858, a metabolically stable triazole antifungal drug, in animals and humans. Antimicrobial Agents Chemother 1985;28:648–53.
26. DeWit S, Weerts D, Goossens H, Clumeck N. Comparison of fluconazole and ketoconazole for oropharingeal candidiasis in AIDS. Lancet 1989;1:746–8.
27. Dupont B, Drouhet E. Fluconazole for the treatment of fungal diseases in immunosuppressed. Am J N Acad Sci 1988;544:564–70.
28. Poland JM. Stomatitis and specific oral infections of the oncologic patients. Am J Hospice Care 1987;Sept/Oct 4:30–32.
29. Lockart PB, Sonis ST. Relationship of oral complications to peripheral blood leukocyte and platelets count in patients receiving cancer chemotherapy. Oral Surgery Oral Med Oral Pathol, 1979;48:21–8.
30. Overholsen CD, Peterson DE, Williams LT et al. Periodontal infections in patients with acute non lymphocytic leukemia: prevalence of acute exacerbations. Arch Int Med 1982;142:551–4.
31. Peterson DE, Overholsen CD. Increased morbidity associated with oral infections in patients with non acute lymphocytic leukemia. Oral Surgery Oral Med Oral Pathol 1981;51:390–3.
32. Minah GE, Rednor JL, Peterson DE et al. Oral succession of Gram-negative bacilli in myelosuppressed cancer patients. J Clin Microbiol 1986;24:210–13.
33. Daeffler R. Oral hygiene measures for patients with cancer I. Cancer Nursing 1980;Oct 3:347–56.
34. Daeffler R. Oral hygiene measures for patients with cancer II. Cancer Nursing 1980;Dec 3:427–32.
35. Regnard C, Fitton S. Mouth care: a flow diagram. Palliat Med 1989;3:67–9.
36. Barret AP. A long term prospective clinical study of orofacial herpes simplex virus infection in acute leukemia. Oral Surgery Oral Med Oral Pathol. 1986;61(2):149–52.
37. Rand HR, Kramer B, Johnson AC. Cancer chemotherapy and associated symptomatic stomatitis and the role of herpes simplex virus. Cancer 1986;50:1262.
38. Barret AP. A long term prospective clinical study of oral complications during conventional chemotherapy for acute leukemia. Oral Surgery Oral Med Oral Pathol 1987;63:313–16.
39. Montgomery RT, Redding SW, Le Maistre CF. The incidence of oral herpes simplex virus infection in patients undergoing cancer chemotherapy. Oral Surgery Oral Med Oral Pathol. 1986;61:238–42.
40. Barret AP, Buckley DJ, Greenberg ML et al. The value of exfoliative cytology in diagnosing of oral herpes infection in immunosoppressed patients. Oral Surgery Oral Med Oral Pathol 1986;62:175–8.
41. Dreizen S, McCredie KB, Keating MJ, Bodey GP. Oral infections associated with chemotherapy in adults with acute leukemia. Postgrad Med 1982;71(6):133–46.
42. Harm JM, Prentice HG, Blacklock HA et al. Acyclovir prophylaxis against herpes virus

infections in severely immunocompromised patients: a randomised double blind study. BMJ 1983;287:384–8.

43. Sheperd IP. The management of the oral complications of leukemia. Oral Surgery Oral Med Oral Pathol 1978;45:543–8.

44. Epstein JB, Sherlock C, Page JL, Spinelli J, Phillips G. Clinical study of herpes simplex virus infection in leukemia. Oral Surgery Oral Med Oral Pathol 1990;70:38–43.

45. Park JB, Park NH. Effect of chlorexidine on the *in vitro* and *in vivo* herpes simplex virus infection. Oral Surgery Oral Med Oral Pathol 1989;67:149–53.

46. Barret AP. Neutropenic ulceration—a distinctive clinical entity. J Periodontol 1987;58(1):51–55.

47. Barret AP. Long term prospective clinical study of neutropenic ulceration in acute leukemia. J Oral Med 1987;42(2):102–5.

48. Sonis ST. Oral complications of cancer therapy. In (ed. Cancerprinciples and practice of oncology, 3rd edn (ed. De Vita VT Jr, Hellman S, Rosenberg SA). Philadelphia: Lippincott, 1989:2144–52.

49. Beck S. Impact of a systematic oral care protocol on stomatitis after chemotherapy. Cancer News 1979;2:185–99.

50. Greenberg MS, Cohen SG, Mckifrick JC et al. The oral flora as a source of septicemia in patients with acute leukemia. Oral Surgery Oral Med Oral Pathol 1982;53:32–6.

51. Lynch MA Ship II. Initial oral manifestations of leukemia. Am Dentistry Assoc 1977;75:932–40.

52. Clark PI, Slevin ML. Allopurinol mouthwash and 5–fluoruracil-induced oral toxicity. Eur J Surg Oncol 1985;11:267–8.

53. Dose AM, Loprinzi CL, Cianflone S et al. A controlled evaluation of an allopurinol mouthwash as prophylaxis against 5–fluoruracil (5–FU)-induced stomatitis: a North Central Treatment Group and Mayo Clinic Study. Proc ASCO 1989;8:341.

54. Reynolds WR, Hickey AJ, Feldman MI. Dental management of the cancer patient receiving radiation therapy. Clin Prevent Dentistry 1980;2:5–9.

55. De Conno F, Ripamonti C, Sbanotto A, Ventafridda V. Oral complications in patients with advanced cancer. J Palliat. Care 1989;5(1):7–15.

56. Bruya MA, Maderia NP. Stomatitis after chemotherapy. Am J Nursing 1975;75:1349–52.

57. Sonis ST, Kunz A. Impact of improved dental services on the frequency of oral complications of cancer therapy for patients with non-head-and-neck malignancies. Oral Surgery Oral Med Oral Pathol 1988;65:19–22.

58. Dudjak LA. Mouth care for mucositis due to radiation therapy. Cancer Nursing 1987;10(3):131–40.

59. Wright WE, Haller JM, Harlow SA, Pizzo PA. An oral disease prevention program for patients receiving radiation and chemotherapy. J Am Dentistry Assoc 1985;110:43–7.

60. Hill HF, Chapman CR, Kornell J, Sullivan K, Saeger L, Benedetti C. Self-administration of morphine in bone-marrow transplant patients reduces drug requirements. Pain 1990;40:121–9.

61. Spielman A, Ben-Aryed H, Gutman D, Szargel R, Deutsch E. Xerostomia-diagnosis and treatment. Oral Med 1981;51(2):144–7.

62. Sreebny LM, Valdini A. Xerostomia. Part I: relationship to other oral symptoms and salivary gland hypofunction. Oral Surgery Oral Med Oral Pathol 1988;66:451–8.

63. Ventafridda V, De Conno F, Ripamonti C, Gamba A, Tamburini M. Quality-of-life assessment during a palliative care programme. Ann Oncol 1990;1:415–20.

64. Twycross RG, Lack SA (ed). Control of alimentary symptoms in far advanced cancer. The mouth. Edinburgh: Churchill Livingstone: New York, 1986:12–39.

65. Chen MS, Daly TE. Xerostomia and complete denture retention. Oral Health 1980; 70:27–9.

66. Tapper-Jones L, Aldred M, Walker DM. Prevalence and intraoral distribution of *Candida albicans* in Sjögren's syndrome. J. Clin Pathol 1980;33:282–7.

67. Markitziu A, Gedalia I, Stabholz A, Shuval J. Prevention of caries progress in xerostomic patients by topical fluoride applications: a study *in vivo* and *in vitro*. J Dentistry 1982;10:248–53.
68. Grad H, Grushka M, Yanover L. Drug-induced xerostomiathe effect and treatment. Can Dentistry Assoc J 1985;4:296–301.
69. Wolff A, Fox PC, Ship JA, Atkinson JC, Macynski AA, Baum BJ. Oral mucosal status and major salivary gland function. Oral Surgery Oral Med Oral Pathol 1990;70:49–54.
70. Zasloff M. Magainins, a class of antimicrobial peptides from *Xenopus* skin: isolation, characterization of two active forms, and partial cDNA sequence of a precursor. Proc Natl Acad Sci USA 1987;84:5449–53.
71. Makkonen TA, Nordman E. Estimation of long-term salivary gland damage induced by radiotherapy. Acta Oncol 1987;26(4):307–12.
72. Anderson MW, Izutsu KT, Rice JC. Parotid gland pathophysiology after mixed gamma and neutron irradiation of cancer patients. Oral Surgery 1981;52:495–500.
73. Brown LR, Dreizen S, Rider I. The effect of radiation-induced xerostomia on saliva and serum lysozyme and immunoglobulin levels. Oral Surgery 1976;41:83–92.
74. Carl W, Schaff NG, Chen TY. Oral care of patients irradiated for cancer of the head and neck. Cancer 1972;30:448–53.
75. Dreizen S, Brown LR, Daly TE, Drane JB. Prevention of xerostomia-related dental caries in irradiated cancer patients. J Dental Res 1977;56:99–104.
76. Eneroth CM, Henrikson CO, Jakobsson PA. Effect of fractionated radiotherapy on salivary gland function. Cancer, 1972;30:1147–53.
77. Wescott WB, Mira JG, Starcke EN, Shannon IL, Thoruby JI. Alterations in whole saliva flow rate induced by fractionated radiotherapy. Am J Roentgenol 1978;130:145–9.
78. Dreizen S, Brown LR, Handler S, Levy BM. Radiation-induced xerostomia in cancer patients. Effect on salivary and serum electrolytes. Cancer 1976;38:273–8.
79. Epstein JB, Schubert MM. Synergistic effect of sialagogoues in management of xerostomia after radiation therapy. Oral Surgery Oral Med Oral Pathol 1987;64:179–82.
80. Cheng VST, Downs J, Herbert D, Aramany M. The function of the parotid gland following radiation therapy for head and neck cancer. Int J Radiat Oncol Biol Phys 1981;7:253–8.
81. Wescott WB, Starcke EN, Shannon IL. Some factors influencing salivary function when treating with radiotherapy. Int J Radiat Oncol Biol Phys 1981;7:535–41.
82. Kuten A, Ben-Aryeh H, Berdicevsky I *et al*. Oral side effects of head and neck irradiation: correlation between clinical manifestations and laboratory data. Int J Radiat Oncol Biol Phys 1986;12:401–5.
83. Shannon IL. Management of head and neck irradiated patients. In Saliva and salivation (ed. Zelles T). Oxford: Pergamon Press, 1981:313–20.
84. Liu RP, Fleming TJ, Toth BB, Keene HJ. Salivary flow rates in patients with head and neck cancer 0.5 to 25 years after radiotherapy. Oral Surgery Oral Med Oral Pathol 1990;70:724–9.
85. Mossman K, Shatzman A, Checharick J. Long-term effects of radiotherapy on taste and salivary function in man. Int J Radiat Oncol Biol Phys 1982;8:991–7.
86. Makkonen TA, Tenovuo J, Vilja P, Heimdahl A. Changes in the protein composition of whole saliva during radiotherapy in patients with oral or pharyngeal cancer. Oral Surgery 1986;62:270–5.
87. Dudiak LA. Mouth care for mucositis due to radiation therapy. Cancer Nursing 1987;10(3):131–40.
88. Carl W. Dental management of head and neck cancer patients. J Surg Oncol 1980;15:265–81.
89. Beumer J, Curtis T, Harrison RE. Radiation therapy of the oral cavity: sequelae and management. Head Neck Surgery 1979;1:301–2.
90. Wescott WB, Starcke EN, Shannon IL. Chemical protection against postirradiation dental caries. Oral Surgery 1975;40:709–19.

91. Heimdahl A, Nord CE. Colonization of oropharynx with pathogenic micro-organisms—a potential risk factor for infection in compromized patients. Chemotherapia 1985;4:186–91.

92. Marks JE, Davis CC, Gottsman VL, Purdy JE, Lee F. The effects of radiation on parotid salivary function. Int J Radiat Oncol Biol Phys 1981;7:1013–19.

93. Crawford JM, Taubman MA, Smith DJ. Minor salivary glands as a major source of secretory immunoglobulin A in the human oral cavity. Science, 1975;190:1206–9.

94. Hensten-Petersen A. Biological activities in human labial and palatine secretions. Arch Oral Biol 1975;20:107–9.

95. Bennett DR, McVeigh S, Rodgers B (ed.) AMA drug evaluations, 5th edn. Chicago: American Medical Association, 1983.

96. Goodman Gilman A, Rall TW, Nies AS, Tylor P (ed.). The pharmacological basis of therapeutics 8th edn. New York: Pergamon Press, 1990.

97. Handelman SL, Baric JM, Espeland MA, Berglund KL. Prevalence of drugs causing hyposalivation in an institutionalized geriatric population. Oral Surgery Oral Med Oral Pathol 1986;62:26–31.

98. Sreebny LM, Valdini A, Yu A. Xerostomia. Part II: relationship to nonoral symptoms, drugs, and diseases. Oral Surgery Oral Med Oral Pathol 1989; 68:419–27.

99. Sreebny LM, Schwartz SS. Reference guide to drugs and dry mouth. Gerodontology 1986;5:75–99.

100. White ID, Hoskin PJ, Hanks GW, Bliss JM. Morphine and dryness of the mouth. BMJ 1989;298:1222–3.

101. Ventafridda V, Ripamonti C, Bianchi M, Sbanotto A, De Conno F. A randomized study on oral morphine and methadone in the treatment of cancer pain. J Pain Symptom Manage 1986;1:203–7.

102. Ventafridda V, Saita L, Barletta L, Sbanotto A, De Conno F. Clinical observations on controlled-release morphine in cancer pain. J. Pain Symptom Manage 1989;4:124–9.

103. Ventafridda V, Tamburini M, Caraceni A, De Conno F, Naldi F. A validation study of the WHO method for cancer pain relief. Cancer 1987;59:850–6.

104. Levine MJ, Aguirre A, Hatton MN et al. Artificial salivas: present and future. J Dental Res 1987;66:693–8.

105. Million RR, Cassini NJ, Clark JR. Cancer of the head and neck. In: Cancer principles and practice of oncology, 3rd edn. (ed. De Vita VT Jr, Hellman S, Rosenberg SA). Philadelphia: Lippincott, 1989:488–590.

106. Rosenblatt HH, Stiehm ER. Long term therapy of chronic mucocutanous candidiasis. Am J Med 1983;74:20–23.

107. Greenspan D. The use of pilocarpine in the irradiation-induced xerostomia. J Dental Res 1979;58:420–3.

108. Fox PC, Van Der Ven PF, Baum BJ, Mandel ID. Pilocarpine for the treatment of xerostomia associated with salivary gland dysfunction. Oral Surgery 1986;61:243–8.

109. Schuller DE, Stevens P, Clausen KP, Olsen J, Gahbauer R, Martin M. Treatment of radiation side effects with oral pilocarpine. J Surg Oncol 1989;42:272–6.

110. Greenspan D. Daniels TE. Effectiveness of pilocarpine in postradiation xerostomia. Cancer 1987;59:1123–5.

111. Epstein JB, Decoteau WE, Wilkinson A. Effect of sialor in treatment of xerostomia in Sjögren's syndrome. Oral Surgery 1983;56:495–9.

112. Papas A. A hydrophillic chewing gum for xerostomic patients. J Dental Res 1979;58: 421–3.

113. Gravenmade EJ, Ronkema PA, Paduers AK. The effect of mucin-containing artificial saliva in severe xerostomia. Int J Oral Surgery 1974;3:435–9.

114. Vergo TJ, Kadish SP. Dentures as artificial saliva reservoirs in the irradiated edentulous cancer patient with xerostomia: a pilot study. Oral Surgery 1981;51:229–33.

115. Hussain M, Kish JA, Crane L et al. The role of infection in the morbidity and mortality of

patients with head and neck cancer undergoing multimodality therapy. Cancer 1991;67:716–21.

116. Barret AP. Metronidazole in the management of anaerobic neck infection on acute leukemia. Oral Surgery Oral Med Oral Pathol 1988;66:287–9.

117. Epstein JG, Stevenson-Moore P. Benzydamine hydrochloride in prevention and management of pain in oral mucositis associated with radiation therapy. Oral Surgery Oral Med Oral Pathol 1988;62:145–8.

118. Twycross RG, Lack SA, (ed.) Control of alimentary symptoms in far advanced cancer. Taste change. Edinburgh: Churchill Livingstone: New York, 1986:57–65.

119. Gray H. Anatomy, descriptive and surgical, 15th edn. New York: Bounty Books, 1977.

120. Guyton AC. Textbook of medical physiology, 5th edn. Philadelphia: Saunders, 1976.

121. Murray RG. Ultrastructure of taste receptors. In Handbook of sensory physiology (ed. Beidler L.M.). New York: Springer-Verlag, 1971:31–5.

122. Schiffman SS. Taste and smell in disease. New Engl J Med 1983;308:1275–9.

123. DeWys WD, Walters K. Abnormalities of taste sensation in cancer patients. Cancer 1975;36:1888–96.

124. Williams LR, Cohen MH. Altered taste thresholds in lung cancer. Am J Clin Nutr 1978;31:122–25.

125. Kashima HK, Kalinowski B. Taste impairment following laryngectomy. Ear Nose Throat J 1979;58:88–92.

126. Mossman KL. Gustatory tissue injury in man: radiation dose response relationship and mechanisms of taste loss. Br J Cancer 1986;53(7S):9–11.

127. Herrmann TH, Adamski K, Stefan M. Storungen von Speichelproduktion und Geschmacksempfindung nach Bestrahlung im oropharyngeal Bereich. Radiobiol Radiother 1984;25:621–9.

128. Mossman KL, Henkin RI. Radiation-induced changes in taste acuity in cancer patients. Int J Radiat Oncol Biol Phys 1978;4:663–70.

129. Willonghby JM. Drug-induced abnormalities of taste sensation. Adverse Drug React Bull 1983;100:368–71.

130. Davies KJT, Musa M, Dormandy TL. Measurements of plasma zinc in malignant disease. J Clin Pathol 1986;21:359–65.

131. Henkin RI, Brandley DF. Hypogeusia corrected by Hi^{++} and Zn^{++}. Life Sci 1970;9:701–9.

132. Henkin RI, Schecter PJ, Hoye R, Mattern C. Idiopathic hypogeusia with dysgeusia, hyposmia and dysosmia: a new syndrome. J Am Med Assoc 1971;217:434–40.

133. Henkin RI. Prevention and treatment of hypogeusia due to head and neck irradiation. J Am Med Assoc 1972;220:870–1.

GENERAL REFERENCES

National Cancer Institute. Consensus development conference on oral complications of cancer therapies: diagnosis, prevention, and treatment. Bethesda, MD:US Department of Health and Human Services, 1990.

Ventafridda V, Ripamonti C, Sbanotto A, De Conno F. Mouth Care. In Oxford textbook of palliative medicine (ed. Doyle D, Hanks GWC, MacDonald N). Oxford Medical Publications: Oxford University Press Inc, New York, 1993:434–47.

4
Asthenia–Cachexia

Hans Neuenschwander and Eduardo Bruera

INTRODUCTION

Cachexia develops in most patients with advanced cancer. It is commonly considered a major contributing cause of death in these patients. (1) Cachexia (derived from the Greek words *kakos* (bad) and *hexis* (condition) is characterized by progressive weight loss and catabolism of host body compartments such as muscle and adipose tissue.

Fatigue and asthenia are recognized as the most frequent symptoms in cancer. Their onset sometimes precedes the diagnosis of malignancy or may be the first manifestation. They may be present during the whole course of the illness and may increase by treatments such as chemotherapy, radiation therapy, or surgery. Asthenia may lead patients to refuse potentially curative treatments. However, in the palliative care setting, it is usually not the target of aggressive assessment and management efforts.

Asthenos (Greek) means absence or loss of strength. Asthenia includes three different major symptoms: fatigue or lassitude defined as easy tiring and decreased capacity to maintain performance, generalized weakness defined as the anticipatory sensation of difficulty in initiating a certain activity, and mental fatigue defined as the presence of impaired mental concentration, loss of memory, and emotional lability. (2) The latter condition is commonly described as the mental status after prolonged mental effort, causing reluctance to retry further efforts. Generalized weakness should be distinguished from localized or regional weakness created by neurological or muscular disorders.

Even more important it seems to us is that cachexia is often a major cause of serious patient discomfort. Other frequent cancer-related symptoms such as pain or nausea have received more attention by investigators in the past 15 years, leading to a consequent improvement in the understanding of assessment and management. The delay in emphasis for cachexia and asthenia may partially explain the lack of recognized standards in assessment and treatment of this frequent symptom complex.

Even though cachexia and asthenia are two conditions that can present independently of one another, there is agreement that in the majority of patients they develop with a strong relationship. In most cases cachexia is probably one of the important etiologic factors of cancer fatigue which in these cases might by considered more as an epi-phenomenon than as a self-standing symptom.

This chapter will give some attention to asthenia as a symptom *per se*. It will underline the complex causality and multidimensional aspects of asthenia, the need for continuous assessment, and give some suggestions on management and future research efforts on this topic. It will specially focus on the relationship between cachexia and asthenia.

SIGNIFICANCE

It is important to distinguish fatigue as a physiological phenomenon accompanying physical effort or a strong intellectual performance from fatigue as a pathological finding. The first can be considered as beneficial and protective against over-exertion. If of reasonable duration, it might also be considered a pleasant feeling. Fatigue as a pathological finding is always a distressing sensation.

In chronic diseases such as malignancy, asthenia serves no beneficial function. No other symptom is perceived as being so closely associated with cancer as asthenia. Therefore, this symptom is often accepted as unavoidable by patients, relatives, and health care professionals. Some palliative care textbooks have suggested that the best approach is to encourage the patient to accept the symptom and learn to live with it. (3) While unfortunately the state of the art may make it necessary for some patients to accept this symptom at the present time, it is important for both care-givers and researchers not to renounce improving knowledge about the mechanisms, assessment, and management of this devastating symptom.

PREVALENCE

Asthenia is universally associated with advanced malignancy. However, there are only a limited number of studies available on the prevalence. Most of these studies focus on patients receiving antineoplastic therapy. The prevalence of asthenia in patients receiving chemotherapy has been estimated to be more than 80% (80–96%). (4) Under radiation therapy, asthenia increases over the course of therapy and can outlast the treatment for months.

A retrospective review of 805 cancer patients found generalized weakness in 40%. (5) Almost half of the patients admitted to St Christopher's Hospice in London complained of weakness. (6) Our group found a prevalence of 75% in patients with terminal cancer. (7) In a prospective study we found asthenia present in 72% of patients with advanced breast cancer. (8)

The frequency of asthenia varies widely in the literature. This variation is partially due to the difference in patient groups (type of tumor, stage, tumor mass, institution, etc.). However, another major reason for this difference is the lack of a 'gold standard' for the definition and assessment of asthenia as discussed below.

As for asthenia, for cachexia the frequency reported in the literature is very variable according to the selection of patient groups. Among 3047 patients enrolled in different ECOG (Eastern Cooperative Oncology Group) studies, in 31% of the patients with malignant lymphoma and in 87% with gastric cancer, cachexia (weight loss of >5% of initial weight in 6 months) was present. (9) Our group found cachexia in 37 out of 72 (51%) advanced cancer patients and in 32 out of 40 (80%) terminally ill patients. (10, 11)

MECHANISMS

In most patients the etiology of asthenia is unknown or, at least, there is no gold standard to define in a proper way one or a few mechanisms relating to this symptom. The main reason is probably the fact that at a given time in a given cancer patient, there are several potential causes of asthenia co-existing (Table 4.1). Asthenia may result from one clearly predominant abnormality or from the sum of a number of less prevalent abnormalities (Fig. 4.1).

Many investigators concorde that cachexia is widely the most frequent and principle cause of asthenia. In a majority of patients asthenia might be more an epi-phenomenon of this wasting syndrome rather than a self-standing feature. Figure 4.2 illustrates the assumed relationship between cachexia and asthenia.

Table 4.1 Causes of asthenia in advanced cancer

Cachexia/malnutrition

Dehydration

Infection (recurrent acute infection, chronic infection as hepatitis, tuberculosis, brucellosis, mononucleosis, herpes, etc.)

Anemia

Chronic hypoxia

Neurologic disorders (autonomic dysfunction, myasthenia syndrome, parkinsonism, demyelinization)

Psychogenic causes

Metabolic and electrolyte disorders

Endocrine disorders (thyreopathy, Morbus Addison, diabetes mellitus, etc.)

Insomnia

Over-exertion (chronic/acute)

Pharmacologic/toxic (narcotics, sedatives, alcohol, chemotherapy, etc.)

Metabolic abnormalities

A number of *metabolic abnormalities* present in cancer patients may interfere with the cachexia–asthenia relationship. Although they are discussed in more detail elsewhere in this book (Chapter 1), we have to remember the importance of focusing on topics such as energy expenditure, fat metabolism, in particular pathologic lipolyses and muscle protein degradation, which are associated with gluconeogenesis.

The available data regarding energy expenditure are controversial. Under physiological conditions the basal metabolic rate decreases in answer to chronic starvation. In malignant disease the findings are still controversial, although there is increasing evidence that at least some patients with advanced tumors present even increased rates of metabolism and energy expenditure compared to control groups with similar weight loss. (12, 13)

An increased rate of gluconeogenesis from amino acids is known and is partially related to the tumor mass. Furthermore on increased Cori cycling, such an energy-consuming mechanism may contribute to a rise in the energy expenses. (14) We can frequently observe glucose intolerance associated with hyperinsulisms.

Free fatty acids and amino acids are the principle products resulting from muscle and adipose tissue catabolism. Although lipids are important substrates for cellular membranes and have an important function as intracellular mediators (eicosanoids and phospholipids) tumors are unable to synthesize their own lipids.

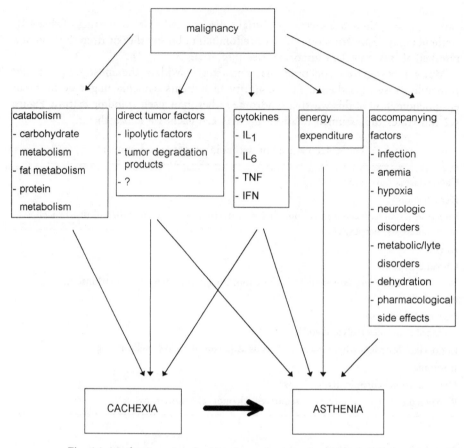

Fig. 4.1 Mechanisms involved in the cachexia-asthenia syndrome.

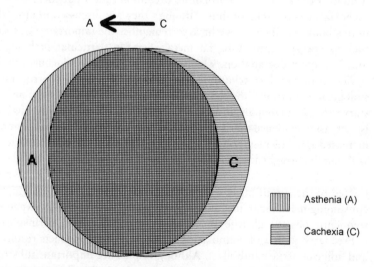

Fig. 4.2 Cachexia-asthenia. Cause and effect—relationship.

Table 4.2 Metabolism in cancer cachexia

Metabolism	Parameters	Finding
Proteins	Nitrogen balance	−
	Whole-body protein synthesis	↑
	Hepatic protein synthesis	↑
	Skeletal muscle protein synthesis	↓
	Skeletal muscle proteolysis	↑
Carbohydrates	Insulin sensitivity	↓
	Gluconeogenesis	↑
	Glucose uptake	↑
	Glycogen stores	↓
Lipids	Serum triglycerides	↑
	Lipoprotein lipase	↑
	Lipogenesis	↓
	Lipolysis	↑
	Total body fat mass	↓
Energy	Energy balance	−
	Energy expenditure	↓↑

From ref. (17).

Nutritional conditions which lead to catabolism of host fat tissue (for example, an acute fast) result in a stimulation of tumor growth suggesting that products from host fat stores may be a limiting factor for tumor growth. (15)

During starvation of healthy subjects a decrease in protein turnover can be observed. (16) Tumor-bearing subjects show an increased requirement for amino acids resulting in a whole body protein breakdown. Cancer cachexia might thus reflect a state of mislead adaptation to a fasting state. Table 4.2 lists the metabolic features found in the presence of cancer cachexia. (17)

More detailed analysis of altered metabolism is treated elsewhere in this book (Chapter 1).

There is some data supporting the hypothesis that wasting is induced by direct catabolism of host components by tumor products, in particular concerning lipid mobilization. (18) On the other hand, cachexia is not strictly dependent on the stage of the tumor and the tumor burden. Indeed it can also be an early effect and simple competition between host and tumor is unlikely to be responsible. An important role is attributed to a number of mediators such as tumor necrosis factor (TNF), interleukin–1 (IL–1), interleukin–6 (IL–6) and interferon (IFN). They are discussed elsewhere in this book (Chapter 1).

As previously discussed, the association between cachexia and asthenia is frequent in cancer patients. Both findings co-exist in the great majority of terminally ill cancer patients. Therefore, it is likely that malnutrition is one of the major contributors to asthenia. (19)

It is proposed that anorexia and asthenia might also be an expression of the major metabolic abnormalities that occur in cancer patients rather than simply an expression of the malnutrition *per se*. (20) This situation would be similar to that experienced when a catabolic state occurs, such as in a viral infection or the early post-operative period. Patients experience anorexia and asthenia in those conditions that are secondary to the metabolic abnormalities and not a cause of those abnormalities.

While the mechanisms of cachexia and anorexia are better understood, the mechanisms of asthenia are much less well known and in some cases asthenia occurs with total independence from cachexia. However, many of the postulated mechanisms for cachexia are applicable to asthenia. Nowadays, it is accepted that the cancer by itself is capable of releasing a number of substances capable of significantly altering the intermediary metabolism of the host. In addition, it is also accepted that the cancer induces the host macrophage to produce and release cachectine and a number of other cytokines (IFN, IL, etc.). It is postulated that for asthenia also there might be a release and/or induction of substances by the tumor. (21, 22) For example, if blood from a fatigued subject is injected into a rested subject, manifestations of fatigue are produced. Tumor-free muscle tissue from tumor-bearing animals shows alterations in the activity of various enzymes, the distribution of isoenzymes, and the synthesis and breakdown of myofibrillar and sarcoplasmic proteins. (21) Some of these hypothetical substances have been termed 'asthenins'.

The muscle and the central nervous system can be considered the main target tissues associated with the perception and expression of asthenia. As mentioned earlier muscle alterations in tumor-bearing patients are well known. Cachexia leads to a loss of muscle mass. This, at least, may partially explain the cachexia-related asthenia. Even in the presence of normal protein and caloric intake and normal body weight, structural and biochemical muscle abnormalities are found in cancer patients. (23–26) Some metabolic abnormalities related to cachexia are specifically responsible for muscle breakdown. Among these, there is an increased concentration of cathepsin–D (a lysosomal enzyme involved in the intracellular degradation of macromolecules). (27) The administration of factors such as eicosapentaenolic acid (EPA) that are capable of inhibiting protein degradation might be an alternative of promise as a therapeutic intervention in these patients. (28)

As mentioned, tumor-bearing patients present muscle abnormalities. Tumor-free muscle tissue of cancer patients shows excessive lactate production. (24) It is unclear whether lactate is part of the pathogenetic mechanism of weakness or just an epiphenomen of it. The atrophy of type II muscle fibers has been suggested to be a systemic effect of cancer even in early and non-metastatic stages. Type II muscle fibers are responsible for high anaerobic glycolytic metabolism. (29) Loss of the contractile machinery of muscle is well known in pathologic processes such as dystrophy, atrophy, inactivity, and metabolic myopathies (treatment with corticosteroids, hypothyroidism, Vitamin D deficiency). In those conditions too there is evidence of atrophy of the type II fibers. One has to establish whether the failure to sustain force is caused by a failure of neural drive (fatigue 'in the mind' or at least in the nervous system rather than in the muscle) (Table 4.3). (30) A proper method of differentiating the two types is represented by a comparison of the force of voluntary and electrically stimulated contractions; another method is the measurement of the muscle temperature rise with force measurement from maximum voluntary and electrically stimulated contractions. (31, 30) Probably in cancer-cachexia-induced fatigue and asthenia both central and peripheral fatigue are involved.

Although there is agreement that cachexia is a major condition leading to asthenia, there may be clinical situations where the relationship is not as close as assumed. To underline and illustrate this hypothesis we may remember that asthenia does occur in non-malignant conditions where malnutrition is absent, such as the chronic fatigue syndrome or psychological depression and also in malignancies that have a low prevalence of malnutrition such as breast cancer or lymphomas. On the other hand, severe malnutrition without asthenia can be observed in patients with anorexia nervosa and in some patient populations with solid tumors.

Table 4.3 Physiological classification of fatigue

Type of fatigue	Definition	Possible mechanism
Central	Force or heat generated by voluntary effort less than that by electrical stimulation.	Failure to sustain recruitment and/or frequency of motor units.
Peripheral	Same force loss or heat generation with voluntary and stimulated contractions.	
– High-frequency fatigue	Selective loss of force at high-stimulation frequency.	Impaired neuromuscular transmission and/or propagation of muscle action potential.
– Low-frequency fatigue	Selective loss of force at low-stimulation frequency.	Impaired excitation–contraction coupling.

From ref. (30).

As illustrated in Fig 4.1 there are a number of tumor-accompanying factors interfering with asthenia such as the following.

Infection

Asthenia often occurs as part of infections, particularly when the course is recurrent or protracted. While it frequently occurs as a prodromic symptom, it may outlast by weeks or months the acute phase of the infection. (32, 33) The presence of immunosuppression increases the risk of infectious complications in cancer patients. Chronic infection and cancer induce the same mediators for cachexia, including cachectine/TNF. (22) It can be hypothesized that they might share similar mediators for asthenia as well.

Anemia

The role of anemia is controversial. While for many years it was thought to be a main cause, recent publications suggest that anemia has been over-valued as a cause of asthenia. In fact, blood supply in anemia cancer patients does not usually result in an improvement of asthenia. However, if the hemoglobin value is extremely low or if the drop has been fast, the correction of anemia might improve the asthenic symptoms. (34)

Neurological changes

There are a number of functional alterations in the midbrain that might be involved in the generation of asthenia. In addition, other neurological syndromes associated with malignancy could be a cause of asthenia. One of them is autonomic dysfunction. This syndrome includes postural hypotension, occasional syncope, fixed heart rate, and gastrointestinal symptoms such as nausea, anorexia, and constipation. (35, 36) The association between autonomic failure and asthenia has not been adequately investigated.

Psychological distress

In patients without cancer who present with asthenia, the final diagnosis is psychologic in almost 75% of cases (depression, anxiety, and other psychological disorders). (37) The prevalence of major psychiatric disorders in cancer patients has been reported to be as low as 2–6%. (38) Other authors have reported a much higher prevalence of psychological abnormalities in cancer patients. (39) In fact, while the clinical experience shows that some depressive symptoms are quite frequent in cancer patients, only a minority of patients develop adjustment disorders and a very small group presents with major depressive or anxiety disorders. (40) The diagnosis of a major depressive episode in the terminally ill patient, although rare, is a major challenge because of the frequent presentation with neurovegetative and somatic symptoms that are part of the disease. The diagnosis should rely more on the presence of psychological and cognitive signs and symptoms. Patients presented with an adjustment disorder or a major depressive disorder can have asthenia as one of the prevalent symptoms. Some authors have found an association between asthenia and mood changes in patients with breast cancer that they had attributed to a combination of the disease and therapy. (41)

Metabolic and endocrine disorders

Disorders such as diabetes mellitus, Addison's syndrome, electrolyte disorders such as low sodium, potassium, or magnesium, and hypercalcemia have to be excluded in particular since some of them have simple and effective treatment.

Over-exertion

This is a frequent cause of asthenia in non-cancer patients. (34) It should be considered also in younger cancer patients who are under aggressive antineoplastic treatment such as radiotherapy and chemotherapy and who are nevertheless trying to maintain their social and professional activity. Research in sports medicine has shown that for prolonged endurance it is important to provide adequate substrate to the muscles (carbohydrate loading). Unfortunately, cancer patients frequently present with abnormalities in muscle metabolism that may not allow for an adequate utilization of this substrate. (36) In addition, recently sports medicine researchers are addressing the role of neurotransmitters such as 5–HT or choline as mediators of fatigue and depression in athletes suffering from over-exertion. (42) Anecdotal evidence suggests that some of these patients' fatigue may disappear after 48 hours of treatment with antidepressants of the 5–HT-specific reuptake inhibitor group. (42) These findings could provide a key to future therapeutic approaches of asthenia.

Side-effects of antineoplastic treatment

Antineoplastic treatments such as surgery, radiation therapy, chemotherapy, and therapy with biological response modifiers are well-known causes of asthenia. The mechanism for asthenia related to all these approaches is not well understood. Specifically, biologic response modifiers are capable of producing a flu-like syndrome. Fatigue becomes the most important dose-limiting side-effects in these patients. In addition to antineoplastic drugs, other drugs administered to patients with advanced cancer can aggravate the level of asthenia. Specifically, opioid agonists such as morphine have significant effects on the reticular system and are capable of inducing sedation, cognitive changes, and asthenia in some patients. In addition, hypnotics are able to cause sedation and asthenia.

Paraneoplastic neurologic syndromes

Although they are rare events, they have to be recognized, since many of these syndromes precede the clinical appearance of a malignancy and they may be partially reversible with a primary treatment of the tumor. Table 4.4 summarizes some of the paraneoplastic neurologic syndromes associated with asthenia. (43)

Table 4.4 Paraneoplastic neurological syndromes associated with asthenia

Progressive multifocal leucoencephalopathy	Leukemia, lymphoma
Paraneoplastic encephalomyelitis	70% lung, 30% others
Amyotrophic lateral sclerosis	
Subacute motor neuropathy	Proximal or distal, often asymmetric (e.g. following irradiated lymphoma)
Subacute necrotic myelopathy	Mostly lung cancer
Peripheral paraneoplastic neurological syndrome	Precedes often the primary, similar to Guillain–Barré
Ascending acute polyneuropathy (Guillain–Barré)	Lymphoma
Neuromuscular paraneoplastic syndromes	
Dermatomyositis, polymyositis	Associated with malignancy in approximately 50% Onset within 1 year
Eaton–Lambert syndrome	Strongly associated with Small cell lung cancer (6%) Can precede tumor by months Improves under successful treatment
Myasthenia gravis	Thymoma (30%), lymphoma

ASSESSMENT

Assessment systems for cancer cachexia are treated elsewhere in this book (Chapter 6). Since asthenia is purely a subjective sensation, it is by nature harder to assess. There is agreement that self-assessment — as in a lot of other symptoms in palliative care — should be the 'gold standard'. The availability of a good and recognized assessment tool is crucial for clinical work and for research purposes. Such an instrument should fullfil the following criteria: simple and not time-consuming aiming at a good compliance over time, enable self-assessment, validity, reliability, and multidimensionality.

Table 4.5 Examples for assessment-tools for asthenia (23)

Unidimensional
  Rhoten Fatigue Scale (44)
  Pearson and Byars Fatigue Feeling Checklist (45)
  Performance status (Karnofsky, ECOG) (46, 47)

Multidimensional
  Fatigue symptom checklist of Kogi, adapted by Kobashi (48)
  Fatigue Self-report Scale (PFS) of Piper (49)
  Edmonton Functional Assessment Tool (EFAT) (50)
  Asthenia-questionnaire proposed by Morant *et al.* (51)

Some proposed assessment tools are listed in Table 4.5. (23) We suggest being familiar with the tool that meets the characteristics of the patient selection and the institutions where one operates. The tool proposed by the group from St Gallen, Switzerland, represents a combination of a questionnaire with a visual analogue scale (VAS). As preliminary results of a small study in 1993, they presented a correlation of asthenia with lack of appetite, anxiety and depression, weight, heart rate, and serum cortisol. However, the proposed questionnaire for evaluation of asthenia in this study was validated in a small sample. The reliability still needs to be confirmed. (51)

Our group has been using the Edmonton Functional Assessment Tool (EFAT) (50) since 1990. This validated instrument assesses asthenia in the context of the functional and performance status of terminally ill patients. Ten items are rated according to predetermined standards of performance which are described in behavioral terms (Table 4.6). These descriptions are ranked from 0 to 3, 0 being independent and 3 being totally dependent. Numerical ratings of the EFAT allow a visual display of performance status, facilitating communication of performance status to the multidisciplinary team.

In our experience, it is simple for the patient and investigator, not very time-consuming, and easy to learn. It has been found to have good values for validity and reliability and it seems to change appropriately according to the changes in the patients clinical status. The use of a numerical scale such as EFAT has the extra advantage of allowing for the adequate measurement of rehabilitative treatment.

Table 4.6 Edmonton Functional Assessment Tool (EFAT)

Items	Rated by
1. Communication	Ability to speak, write, read, and use communication devices
2. Pain	Extent of limitation to participate in desired activity by physical suffering
3. Mental status	Self, place, time; recall immediate, recent, remote events respond and follow instructions
4. Dyspnea	Degree to which shortness of breath limits participation in desired activity
5. Balance	Ability to maintain and regain sitting or standing position
6. Mobility	Ability to move, attaining sitting from side lying, transfers from bed to chair
7. Walk/wheelchair locomotion	
8. Activities of daily living (ADL)	Wash, dress, comb hair, brush teeth, use toilet, feed oneself
9. Fatigue	Subjective feeling of weariness, weakness, exhaustion, lack of energy resulting from prolonged stress
10. Motivation	Ability to initiate movement or behaviour, induces a person to act, desire
Performance status	Overall judgment of functional performance

MANAGEMENT

Weight loss and wasting are common adverse effects of malignancy. They can occur early in the course of the illness. They might usually be preceded for months or even years by subclinical alterations in the different metabolic mechanisms, since clinical evidence of cachexia has to be considered an 'end-stage' of this important effect. To understand the cachexia-inducing mechanisms is therefore a mandatory condition in developing the key to reverse or even prevent it.

Unfortunately the experimental models dealing with the study of cachexia mechanisms usually do not fullfil the criteria that cachexia should be an early effect of tumor. The few exceptions show that weight loss can be present without evidence of loss of appetite. (52, 53)

It is therefore unlikely, that a simple competition between host and tumor is responsible for cachexia and for cachexia-related asthenia.

Although malnutrition can cause abnormal muscle function, (54) there is no established evidence that nutritional therapy is an important key to subjective improvement. Thus, asthenia alone is not an indication for generalized aggressive nutritional treatment of cancer patients.

Since asthenia is a complex, multi-dimensional symptom, it is crucial for an adequate therapeutic approach to identify and prioritize the different underlying factors. It is clear that in this attempt, prior experience and personal bias will play a significant role. The change of asthenia over time may allow a stronger association with a particular finding (for example, is an increase in asthenia following the same progression as a growth in the tumor size, an increase in the serum calcium, or a change in the drug treatment?).

In planning the therapeutic approach it is also important to answer the following questions.

1. Is, for a given patient, asthenia a symptom of primary importance?

2. What are the major probable causes?

3. Are there therapeutic measures available with a reasonable cost–benefit ratio?

The intervention may have the purpose of either decreasing the intensity of asthenia or allowing the patient to express the maximal possible level of function with a stable level of asthenia, or both. Figure 4.3 summarizes some of general and specific measure that can be pursued.

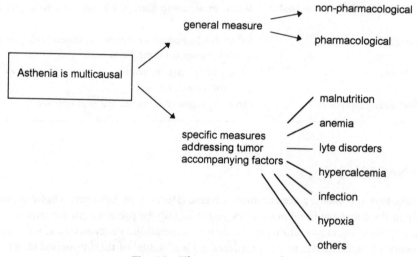

Fig. 4.3   Therapeutic approach

General measures

Non-pharmacological measures

It is crucial to keep the patient informed about his/her status, the causes of the loss of energy, and the type of therapeutic options available, in order to avoid an information gap and to allow the patient the opportunity to develop realistic expectations.

If patients are empowered by the correct information and counseling they may combat asthenia as follows.

1. Adapting activities of daily living. (For example, decreasing housework and allowing help with physical duty).

2. Rearranging time schedules during the day.

3. Spending more time in bed.

4. Requesting changes in medications perceived as causing loss of energy.

5. Avoiding particularly energy-expending activities. (55)

The care givers must try to find a balance between 'more rest' which is capable of decreasing the intensity of asthenia and increased deconditioning thereby inducing further weakness.

Fatigue can be a side-effect of exercise (over-exertion). More frequently it might develop as a result of inappropriatness of exercise. If a patient complains of fatigue while performing moderate exercise the proper intervention is to stop it. Moderate exercise is generated by type I fibers (low myosin-ATPase activity). Type I fibers (implicated in activities such as aerobic performance of low strength, for example maintenance of posture) are typically highly resistant to fatigue.

Exercise is at the beginning followed by decreased protein synthesis and increased protein catabolism. At a certain point, however, these effects are reversed, leading to growing muscle mass. (56)

The time course of these events is unclear and has to be established. There are indications that in an early stage of cachexia moderately forced exercise might be beneficial while in an advanced stage exercise that exceeds spontaneous physical activity might cause more harm than good. (57)

Pharmacological measures
In patients with asthenia of unknown origin or in those in whom a specific treatment is not available, a number of non-specific pharmacological interventions have been proposed.

Corticosteroid These drugs have been suggested by a number of studies to be able to decrease asthenia in cancer. In addition to anecdotal reports, (54) controlled randomized trials have confirmed the presence of decreased asthenia. The level of activity and the final blinded choice of patients and investigators were able to identify methylprednisolone at 32 mg/day as more effective than a placebo. In this report, however, the duration of the effect was limited to 2–3 weeks. (58)

The mechanism of action of steroids on asthenia is unknown. Both the inhibition of tumor-induced substances as well as a central euphoriant effect are potential mechanisms.

While there is agreement on the positive short-term effect of steroids on physical and mental performance and the mood, metabolic side-effects have to be taken into account. Steroids lead to a series of mechanisms with a potential paradoxical effect on performance (increased gluconeogenesis, catabolic activities, immunologic depression, and, last but not least, the steroid myopathy, that occurs, however, usually after 2–3 months of therapy). Therefore steroids might have a good effect in short-term use; in a longer treatment (for example, in patients with a less limited life expectancy), the negative effects of steroids could overwhelm.

Amphetamines In 1977 Forrest *et al.* (59) reported improved cognition and decreased sedation in post-operative patients receiving dextro-amphetamine. (59) In an open study, 16 advanced cancer patients were treated with dextro-amphetamine, of whom 12 appeared to experience improvement in activity. (60) Our group studied mazindol in a double-blind, placebo-controlled study in patients with advanced cancer. (61) This drug was found to have some positive effect on pain, but no significant effect on asthenia. In addition, significant neurotoxicity occurred. In a follow-up study, methylphenidate (a mild short-acting amphetamine derivate) was given to patients receiving higher doses of opioids. In this 3-day, double-blind cross-over study, methylphenidate appeared to improve asthenia compared to a placebo. Our experience with methylphenidate and mazindol suggests that these drugs would be useful exclusively in those patients in whom asthenia results from increasing doses of opioids and not in order to improve general 'well-being'. The use of amphetamine derivate has been proposed for patients presenting with hypoactive, hypoalert delirium. (62)

Since asthenia was not the main outcome measurement of any of the trials on amphetamine, it is not possible to establish whether these drugs have a true effect on asthenia or if it is a question of improvement of other symptoms that co-exist in this patient population.

Evaluating the usefulness of an amphetamine prescription to treat asthenia we need to consider also the negative potential of anorexia which is potentially induced by these drugs, therefore in the longer term they may contribute to the malnutrition.

Large attention has been given to Megesterol acetate (MEA). In a number of studies the positive effect on cachexia in cancer and AIDS populations has been evidenced. Weight gain is not only limited to water retention but due also to stimulation of lipocytes. This drug is so far the most effective available in the pharmacological treatment of cachexia. It may be justified to argue whether this is also due to the encouragement of the pharmaceutical industry to run trials on MEA. Since MEA is expensive and the segment of patients that could potentially benefit is large, randomized trials with MEA versus for example corticosteroids, not just with weight gain and other anthropometric parameters, but with quality of life items as end-points, are urging. The positive effect of MEA on cachexia is established and a direct effect of MEA on asthenia has been reported but needs further confirmation. (63)

Details on MEA trials are treated elsewhere in this book (Chapter 9).

Specific measures

As previously discussed, asthenia is often multicausal. It may appear as an epiphenomenon of other symptom complexes such as those related to cachexia, infection, anemia, etc., rather than as a self-standing single issue. Any measure able to reverse the underlying abnormality would result in an improvement in asthenia. It is useful to represent graphically the proportional participation of different reasons with the aim of identifying reversible partial causes. Reversible causes such as dehydration, metabolic disorders, or severe anemia may co-exist with non-reversible causes. The list of prescribed drugs must be continuously checked to avoid asthenia as an iatrogenic effect (for example, accumulation of opioids in the presence of renal failure). Psychological reasons such as depression, anxiety, and over-exertion can be therapeutically addressed. The treatment of malnutrition as a cause of asthenia in the specific situation of cancer patients remains controversial. Malnourished patients are known to have a significant level of asthenia. However, once cachexia is established it has not been clearly demonstrated that attempts to reverse the level of malnutrition are able to result in any significant improvement in the level of asthenia. (64, 65) It might be different when we address malnutrition in an early, subclinical stage. One could imagine that nutritional support, including in particular nutritional adjuncts such as vitamins and trace elements, offered preventively could avoid cachexia and cachexia-related asthenia. So far it is mandatory to define standards to establish early stages of malnutrition and introduce them in a clinical routine. Oncologists must use them as a daily instrument and conduct trials to determine whether earlier attention in the course of the disease is able to avoid or decrease the level of asthenia.

In palliative care the satisfactory treatment of a symptom such as asthenia does not mean that it is mandatory to eliminate it completely. Even minor improvements would be enough to shift asthenia into a less relevant level in the patient's priority symptom list. Figure 4.4 summarizes the case of a 60-years-old man with metastatic non-small cell lung cancer, who was complaining of severe asthenia. The patient had lost 6 kg in four months and had developed two pneumonias in the previous 3 months. His oxygen saturation was 84%, his hemoglobin was 11.5 g % and he was clinically dehydrated. He was currently receiving therapy with 180 g morphine parenterally every 24 hours. He was also receiving Lorazepam at night because of insomnia. The approach in this patient included the elimination of the toxic effects of opioids by switching from morphine to another active opioid and rehydration. These changes were able to decrease the intensity of asthenia in the visual analog scale from 85 to 55. At that time, other symptoms such as shortness of breath became more important than asthenia.

VAS for asthenia / fatigue

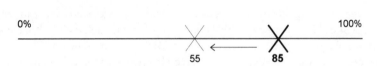

causes of asthenia	estimated percentage	not easily treatable	easily treatable
malnutrition	45%	X	
post infection	10%	X	
hypoxia	5%		X
dehydration	10%		X
opioids (accumulation)	15%		X

Fig. 4.4 Sixty-year-old man with metastatic NSCLC. Weight loss, recurrent infections, dehydration, hypoxia, impaired renal function. Therapy: antibiotic, narcotic, hypnotic.

Future research

While cancer cachexia has been addressed by research in the last decade, knowledge about asthenia is limited and research in this field is still in its infancy. Progress on this topic since this symptom affects almost every patient is urgent; thus we will mention some suggestions for future research.

1. Awareness must take place that asthenia is a symptom of high prevalence, thus it is unacceptable that it is just to consider irreversible.

2. In order to speak a common language among scientists and clinicians a valid and reliable tool for assessment is needed.

3. The association between malnutrition and asthenia is well recognized in cancer and geriatric patients. However, aggressive nutrition has not been proven to improve asthenia significantly in cancer patients. Malnourished patients without cancer frequently benefit from substances such as vitamins and trace elements. Cancer patients frequently present with a number of nutritional deficiencies. The role of some specific nutrients on asthenia should be better established.

4. There are only preliminary studies on the benefit of exercise on asthenia. No conclusions can be drawn so far. Since exaggerated exercise might induce or maintain fatigue, anticipatory fatigue might lead to avoidance. This anticipation may be due to just one or few negative experiences in particular when started in a too enthusiastic manner. Prospective studies are needed in the area of activity rest. How much rest is beneficial? Is the fear of deconditioning justified? At what level is physical activity leading to counter-productive exertion?

5. The role of drugs such as megestrol acetate, corticosteroids, and anabolic steroids should be better established. Some of them such as MPA have shown evidence of a positive effect on cancer and AIDS-related cachexia. All these drugs have been anecdotally suggested to have effects on asthenia in cancer patients. However, since these findings have consistently not been the main outcome measurements of studies, it is difficult to establish a role for any of these pharmacological interventions in the management of asthenia.

REFERENCES

1. Lawson DH, Richmond A, Nixon DW, Rudman D. Metabolic approaches to cancer cachexia. Ann Rev Nutr 1982;2:277–301.
2. Theologides A. Asthenia in cancer. Am J Med 1982;73:1–3. Bruera E, MacDonald RN. Asthenia in patients with advanced cancer. J Pain Symptom Manage 1988;3(1):9–14.
3. Saunders C. The management of terminal malignant disease, 2nd ed. London: Edward Arnold, 1989.
4. Irvine DM, Vincent L, Bubela N, Thompson L, Graydon J. A critical appraisal of the research literature investigating fatigue in the individual with cancer. Cancer Nursing 1991;14(4)188–99.
5. Lehman J, De Lisa J, Warren C et al. Cancer rehabilitation: assessment of need, development and evaluation of a model care. Arch Phys Med Rehabil 1978;59:410–19.

6. Walsh T, Saunders C. Hospice care: the treatment of pain in advanced cancer. Recent Results in Cancer Res 1984;89:201–11.
7. Bruera E, MacDonald RN. Asthenia in patients with advanced cancer. J Pain Symptom Manage 1988;3(1):9–14.
8. Bruera E, Brenneis C, Michaud M, Jackson F, MacDonald RN. Association between involuntary muscle function (IMF) and asthenia (AST), nutritional status (NS), lean body mass (LBM), psychometric assessment and tumor mass (TM) in patients (PTS) with advanced breast cancer. Proc Am Soc Clin Oncol 1987;6:261.
9. De Wys WD, Begg C, Lavin et al. Prognostic effect of weight loss prior to chemotherapy in cancer patients. Am J Med 1980;69:491–7.
10. Bruera E, Roca E, Carraro S. Association between malnutrition and caloric intake, emesis psychological depression, anxiety, appetite and activity in terminal cancer patients. Cancer Treat Rep 1986;70:295–8.
11. Bruera E, Roca E, Cedaro L, Carraro S, Chacon R. Action of oral methylprednisolone in terminal cancer patients: a prospective randomized doubleblind study. Cancer Treat Rep 1985;69:751–4.
12. Legapsi A, Jeevanadam M, Starnes HF, Brennan MF. Whole body lipid and energy metabolism in the cancer patient. Metabolism 1987;10:958–63.
13. Nelson KA, Walsh D, Sheehan FA. The cancer anorexia–cachexia syndrome. JCO 1994;12(1):213–25.
14. Douglas RG, Shaw JHF. Metabolic effects of cancer. Br J Surgery 1990;77:246–54.
15. Tisdale MJ. Cancer cachexia. Br J Cancer 1991;63:337–42.
16. Rose D, Horowitz GD, Jeevanadam M, Brennan MF, Shives GT, Lowry SF. Whole body protein kinetics during acute starvation and intravenous refeeding in normal man. Fed Proc 1983;42:1070.
17. Pisters PWT, Pearlstone DB. Protein and amino acid metabolism in cancer cachexia: investigative techniques and therapeutic interventions. Crit Rev Clin 1993;30(3):223–72.
18. Beck SA, Tisdale MJ. Lipid mobilising factors specifically associated with cancer cachexia. BR J Cancer, 1991;63:846–50.
19. Bruera E. Current pharmacological management of anorexia in cancer patients. Oncology 1992;6(1):125–30.
20. Bruera E. Clinical management of cachexia and anorexia in patients with advanced cancer. Oncology 1992;49(Suppl 2):35–42.
21. Theologides A. Asthenins and cachectins in cancer. Am J Med 1986;81:696–8.
22. Beutler B, Cerami A. Cachectin: more than a tumor necrosis factor. New Engl J Med 1987;316(7):379–85.
23. Neuenschwander H, Bruera E. Asthenia in cancer patients. In: Oxford textbook of palliative medicine 2nd ed. (ed. Doyle D, Hanks E, MacDonald N) Oxford Medical Publications, in press.
24. Holroyde R, Axelrod RS, Skutchers CL, Haff AC, Paul P, Reichard SA. Lactate metabolism in patients with metastatic colorectal cancer. Cancer Res 1979;39:4900–4.
25. Beck S, Mulligan H, Tisdale M. Lipolytic factors associated with murine and human cancer cachexia. J Natl Cancer Inst 1990;82:1922–6.
26. Smith KL, Tisdale MJ. Mechanism of muscle protein degradation in cancer cachexia. Br J Cancer 1993;68:314–18.
27. Beck SA, Tisdale MJ. Production of lipolytic and proteolytic factors by a murine tumor producing cachexia in the host. Cancer Res 1987;47:5919–23.
28. Beck SA, Smith KL, Tisdale MJ. Anticachectic and antitumor effect of eicosapentaenolic acid and its effect on protein turnover. Cancer Res 1991;51:6089–93.
29. Warmolts JR, Re PK, Lewis RJ, Engel WK. Type II muscle fibre atrophy (II–Atrophy): an early sistemic effect of cancer. Neurology 1975;2:374.
30. Edwards RHT. New techniques for studying human muscle function, metabolism and fatigue. Muscle Nerve 1984;7:599–609.

31. Edwards RHT. Physical analysis of skeletal muscle weakness and fatigue. Clin Sci 1978;54:463–70.
32. Jones J, Ray G, Minnich L. Evidence for active Epstein–Barr virus infection in patients with persistent, unexplained illnesses: elevated anti-early antigen antibodies. Ann Int Med 1985;102:1–7.
33. Strauss S, Tosato G, Armstrong G et al. Persistent illness and fatigue in adults with evident Epstein–Barr virus infection. Ann of Int Med 1985;102:7–16.
34. Plum F. Asthenia, weakness and fatigue. In Wyngaarden J, Smith L, editors. Cecil textbook of medicine. Philadelphia: Saunders, 1985:2044.
35. Henrich W. Autonomic insufficiency. Arc Int Med 1982;9–44.
36. Bruera E, Chadwick S, MacDonald N, Fox R, Hanson J. Study of cardiovascular autonomic insufficiency in advanced cancer patients. Cancer Treat Rep 1986;70(12):1383–7.
37. Adams R. Anxiety, depression, asthenia and personality disorders. In: Harrison's principles of internal medicine (ed. Petersdorf R, Adams R, Braunwald E. New York: McGraw-Hill, 1983; 68–75.
38. Derogatis L, Morow G, Fetting J et al. The prevalence of psychiatric disorders among cancer patients. J Am Med Assoc 1983;249:751–7.
39. Breitbart W, Pasnik SD. Psychiatric aspects of palliative care. In: Oxford textbook of palliative medicine. (ed. Doyle D, Hanks G, MacDonald N). London: Oxford Medical Publications, 1993;609–26.
40. Hayes JR. Depression and chronic fatigue in cancer patients. Primary Care 1991;18(2):327–39.
41. Piper BF. Fatigue. Trans-culturale implications for nursing interventions. Presented at the Sixth International Conference on Cancer Nursing, Amsterdam 1990.
42. Burfoot A. The brain connection. Runners World 1994;29(8):70–5.
43. Warenius HM. Paraneoplastic neurological syndromes. In The Clinical Neurology of old Age. (ed. Tallis, R). John Wiley, 1989:323–34.
44. Rhoten D. Fatigue and postsurgical patient. In Norris CM, (edition) Concept clarification in nursing. Rockville, MD: Aspen Publisher 1982;277–300.
45. Pearson PG, Byars GE. The development and validation of a checklist measuring subjective fatigue. Report no. 556115. School of Aviation, USAF, Randolf AFB, Texas, 1956.
46. Stanley K. Prognostic factors for survival in patients with inoperable lung cancer. J Natl Cancer Inst 1980;65:25–32.
47. Minna J, Higgins G, Glastein E. Cancer of the lung. In: Cancer principles and practice of oncology (ed. De Vita V, Hellman S, Rosenberg S). New York; Lippincott, 1982:434.
48. Kobashi-Schoot JAM, Hanewald GJFP, van Dam FSAM et al. Assessment of malaise in cancer treated with radiotherapy. Cancer Nursing 1985;8:306–14.
49. Piper BF Lindsey AM, Dodd MJ et al. The development of an instrument to measure the subjective dimension of fatigue. In: (ed. Key aspects of comfort. Management of pain, fatigue and nausea. Funk S, Tornquist E, Compagne M, Gopp L, Wiese C). New York: Springer Publishing Co, 1989:199–208.
50. Kaasa T, Gillis K, Middleton E, Bruera E. The Edmonton Functional Assessment Tool (EFAT) for terminal cancer patients. Presented at the 9th International Congress on Care of the Terminally Ill, Montreal, Nov. 1–2, 1992.
51. Morant R, Stiefel F, Berchtold W, Radziwill A, Riesen W. Preliminary results of a study assessing asthenia and related psychological and biological phenomena in patients with advanced cancer. Supp Care Cancer 1993;1(2):101–7.
52. Bibby MC, Double JA, Ali SA, Fearon KC, Brennan RA, Tisdale MJ. Characterisation of a transplantable adenocarcinoma of the mouse colon producing cachexia in recipient animals. J Natl Cancer Inst 1987;78:539–46.
53. Tanaka Y, Eda H, Tanaka T et al. Experimental cancer cachexia induced by transplantable colon 26 adenocarcinoma in mice. Cancer Res 1990;50:2290–5.

54. Lopes J, Russell D, Whitwell J et al. Skeletal muscle function in malnutrition. Am J Clin Nutr 1983;36:602–10.
55. Love R, Leventhal H, Easterling M, Nerenz D. Side effects and emotional distress. Cancer 1989;63:604–12.
56. Dohm L, Kasperek GJ, Tapscott EB, Beecher GR. Effect of exercise on synthesis and degradation of muscle protein. Biochem Med 1982; 27:254–9.
57. Daneryd PLE, Hafström LR, Karlberg IH. Effects of spontaneous physical exercise on experimental cancer anorexia and cachexia. Eur J Cancer 1990;26(10):1083–8.
58. Bruera E, Cararro S, Roca E et al. Double blind evaluation or mazindol in enhancing the comfort of terminally ill cancer patients. Cancer Treat Rep 1986;71:67–70.
59. Forrest W, Brown B, Brown C et al. Dextroamphetamine with morphine for the treatment of post-operative pain. New Engl J Med 1977;296:712–5.
60. Weiner N. Amphetamine. In: The pharmacological basis for therapeutics (ed. Goodman L, Gilman A). New York: Macmillan, 1980; 159–62.
61. Bruera E, Roca E, Cedaro L, Carraro S, Chacon R. Action of oral methylprednisolone in terminal cancer patients: a prospective randomized double-blind study. Cancer Treat Rep 1985;69(7/8):751–4.
62. Bruera E, Brenneis C, Chadwick S. Methylphenidate associated with narcotics for the treatment of cancer pain. Cancer Treat Rep 1987;71:67-70.
63. Bruera E, MacMillan K, Kuehn N, Hanson J, MacDonald RN, A controlled trial of megestrol acetate of appetite, caloric intake, nutritional status and other symptoms in patients with advanced cancer. Cancer 1990;66:1279–82.
64. Kortez R. Parenteral nutrition: is it oncologically logical? J Clin Oncol 1984;2:534–8.
65. Evans W, Nixon D, Daly J. A randomized study of standard or augmented oral nutritional support versus ad lib nutrition intake in patients with advanced cancer. Clin Invest Med 1986;9:A–127 (Abstract).

5

Clinical epidemiology of cancer cachexia

Robert Dunlop

INTRODUCTION

The diagnosis of cancer is still feared by the lay public. It is a common illness which causes almost 25% of all deaths. (1) Although the prospect of a painful agonizing death is the most worrying, the gaunt appearance of people with advanced cancer also has a vivid association in the minds of the public. This association is an indication of how frequently cachexia occurs.

There are several problems in estimating the prevalence of the cachexia–anorexia syndrome. The syndrome is well recognized and well defined. However, symptoms such as loss of appetite and loss of weight can have multiple causes including the paraneoplastic effects of cancer, the effects of cancer treatments, and concurrent non-malignant conditions which produce malnutrition (see Chapter 1). The studies of cachexia rarely differentiate between these causes.

The other major problem relates to sampling. Most studies have been conducted in medical or surgical wards, oncology services, or hospices. Each of these settings caters for a subset of cancer patients and conclusions from any one, or indeed from all, cannot be generalized. Several studies have used random sampling of death certificates to provide population-based information on the last year of life. These studies rely on the memories of relatives which may not accurately reflect the experience of the patients. (2) In addition, the patients who survive as a result of treatment and the patients without respondents are not sampled by this means.

Bearing the above problems in mind, this chapter will review the incidence of cachexia with respect to primary tumor, disease stage, patient characteristics, and antineoplastic treatments. The effects of cachexia on the response to anticancer treatments will also be considered.

THE INCIDENCE OF CACHEXIA IN CANCER PATIENTS

The reported incidence of cachexia varies widely. One reason for this variation relates to the point in the cancer history when patients are studied. In their review of nutrition in cancer patients, Bruera and MacDonald (3) contrasted the low proportion of patients (2.3%) with malnutrition who were receiving adjuvant chemotherapy with the majority of patients who were malnourished with terminal cancer (80%).

At the time of recruitment into chemotherapy trials, weight loss was apparent in 54% of 3047 patients seen by the Eastern Cooperative Oncology Group (ECOG). (4) Three studies (5–7) found that 51, 60, and 66% respectively, of patients with cancer of the stomach, oesophagus, pancreas, and colon/rectum had significant weight loss and other evidence of malnutrition prior to operation.

Curtis (8) measured 38 symptoms of 100 patients presenting to a palliative care service within a tertiary referral centre. Weight loss was present in 58% of patients and anorexia in 55%. Dunlop (9) found a similar incidence of anorexia (58%) in 50 patients with advanced cancer in hospice and hospital settings. At St Christopher's Hospice (SCH), 79% of 608 terminally ill patients reported weight loss during the routine symptom assessment conducted on admission. Coyle *et al.* (10) found a much lower prevalence (8%) of loss of appetite in 90 patients with advanced cancer. However, they only recorded symptoms which patients spontaneously reported as being distressing enough to interfere with activity and studied patients admitted to an American cancer centre. Brescia *et al.* (11) also found a much lower prevalence of anorexia in 1103 patients with advanced cancer admitted to an acute hospital. However, the presence or absence of the symptom was determined retrospectively from case records. The lower prevalence in these last two reports may be due to the earlier stages of illness in patients seen by cancer centres compared with palliative care services.

The Regional Study of the Care of Dying, based on a random sample of deaths in 20 health districts in England, found that 78% of 2051 cancer patients experienced a lack of appetite, in the opinion of the surviving relatives. This figure compares with 44% of the 1581 patients with non-malignant conditions sampled in the same study (Addington-Hall J, written communication). One-third of cancer patients who died experienced anorexia for more than 6 months, while 43% were anorexic for 1–6 months. Only half of the anorexic patients were deemed by the relatives to have been distressed by loss of appetite. This fact should be borne in mind when talking with terminally ill patients and their relatives about loss of appetite. Relatives are often more worried about anorexia or the patient will be concerned because the relatives are worried (see Chapter 12). In this situation, it is more appropriate to reassure the carers on behalf of the patient. Reassurance is more successful when coupled with practical advice which helps allay the family's sense of helplessness, such as serving small meals on small plates.

PRIMARY TUMOR AND CACHEXIA

The frequency of weight loss varies according to the primary diagnosis. Dewys *et al.* (4) studied 11 diagnosis groups and the frequency of weight loss varied from 31% in patients with non-Hodgkins lymphoma to 87% of patients with gastric cancer. It might be expected that the ECOG data could underestimate the frequency of weight loss because cachectic patients would be less likely to be referred for chemotherapy. However, their data suggest that the frequency of cachexia is higher for patients with solid tumors compared with haematological malignancies. The main exception among solid tumors is breast cancer, which maintains normal nutrition until late in the natural history of the illness. In late-stage illness, a study of 608 cancer patients who died within six weeks of admission to St Christopher's Hospice, found that differences in the frequency of weight loss were less apparent (Table 5.1). In this group, weight loss was less likely with breast cancer and colon cancer.

Table 5.1 Comparison of weight loss in terminally ill patients versus patients referred for chemotherapy

Diagnosis	SCH data Number of patients	% with weight loss	ECOG data Number of patients	% with weight loss
Lung cancer	147	89	1026	57–61
Breast cancer	66	53	289	36
Colon cancer	76	75	307	54
Prostate cancer	44	89	78	56
Pancreas cancer	22	82	111	83
Gastric cancer	25	87	317	87
Unknown primary	31	94	–	–
Lymphoma	7	86	601	31–48
Overian cancer	20	95	–	–
Oesophagus cancer	25	96	–	–
Total (including other diagnoses)	608	79	3047	54

The variability in weight loss is difficult to explain, particularly in the absence of data on previous treatment and other contributory factors. The potential effects of anticancer treatments will be examined later in the chapter. Some cancers produce direct effects which cause weight loss. Head and neck cancers can interfere with swallowing by a mass effect or by damaging cranial nerves. Oesophageal and intra-abdominal malignancies may cause obstruction. Malabsorption may be associated with pancreatic cancer. However, these direct effects cannot explain weight loss in most patients; distant paraneoplastic effects of cancer have been implicated. The experimental evidence for paraneoplastic metabolic abnormalities is reviewed in the chapter on the pathophysiology of cachexia in advanced cancer and AIDS (see Chapter 1).

CACHEXIA AND DISEASE STAGE

The ECOG study examined the relationship between the extent of the cancer and the presence of weight loss. (4) The tumor extent was defined by the involvement of liver, lungs, or bone. The authors noted that the score derived from this definition could not be equated with the total tumor volume. Breast cancer patients with two or three organs involved were statistically more likely to have significant weight loss compared with patients with no or one organ involved (49% versus 31%). Patients with sarcoma or colon cancer with two or more organs involved also had a greater than 10% increase in frequency of weight loss but this was not statistically significant. There was no association for patients with prostate, lung, pancreas, or gastric cancer. Other authors have failed to demonstrate a link between disease stage and weight loss.

PATIENT CHARACTERISTICS AND CACHEXIA

In our review of over 600 patients dying in St Christopher's Hospice, there was no difference in the frequency of weight loss according to age or sex. Curtis (8) also found no gender difference in the incidence of weight loss but anorexia and early satiety occurred more frequently in women. Women were also more likely to relate these symptoms as severe but this difference did not reach statistical significance. Older patients may be somewhat less likely to experience anorexia. Seale and Cartwright (12) found that 58% of patients over the age of 75 years experienced loss of appetite compared with 77% of younger patients. However, Brescia *et al.* (11) did not find any difference in the proportion of patients with anorexia under 65 years of age compared with older patients. The limitation of this data has already been described in this chapter. Dewys *et al.* (4) noted that weight loss was associated with a reduction in performance status except in patients with pancreatic and gastric cancer.

ANTINEOPLASTIC TREATMENTS AND CACHEXIA

Chemotherapy may cause weight loss by a variety of mechanisms. (13) Nausea and vomiting are side-effects which depend on the dose and type of medication. Cisplatinum, dacarbazine, nitrogen mustard, and intravenous cyclophosphamide are particularly likely to cause emesis, while daunorubicin, doxorubicin, carmustine, and procarbazine are examples of drugs with a moderate emetogenic potential. A wide range of anti-emetic drugs are available to minimize these effects. The recently introduced 5–HT receptor antagonists have been particularly effective, to the extent that dacarbazine, for example, is being reconsidered by oncologists who had abandoned its use. Even in the absence of nausea, patients can become debilitated by the more insidious loss of appetite which can respond to anti-emetic therapy.

Chemotherapy can also affect the mouth causing painful ulceration and infection. This will lead patients to avoid eating and swallowing. Aggressive mouth care and appropriate use of analgesics can minimize these effects. Dose reduction of the chemotherapy agents may be necessary if stomatitis is related to neutropenia. In some cases, chemotherapy-induced damage to the epithelial surface of the small bowel will impair absorption but the clinical effects are minimal. (13) This is discussed in more detail in Chapter 3.

The effects of chemotherapy on weight loss have been quantified. Samuels *et al.* (14) compared vinblastine and bleomycin with vinblastine, bleomycin, and cisplatin. Both groups lost weight with a mean loss of 4.19 versus 5.60 kg per course, respectively. The maximum weight loss occurred after the first course (5.94 versus 8.70 kg). Another study of multiagent chemotherapy for patients with small cell lung cancer described a median post-therapy weight loss of 3.6 kg. (15)

Radiotherapy can also cause weight loss, depending on the site which is irradiated and the dose which is delivered. Anorexia, nausea, and vomiting can occur if the bowel lies within the radiotherapy field. Painful mucositis frequently follows treatment of the mouth or oesophagus. These acute effects are usually temporary.

Some of the late effects of radiotherapy will cause weight loss. Chronic inflammation of the gut may ensue, associated with diarrhoea and malabsorption. The changes induced by end-arteritis will cause fibrosis, stricturing, ulceration, fistula formation, or perforation of the bowel. These late effects are frequently mistaken for the effects of advanced cancer. A high degree of suspicion must be maintained so that the correct diagnosis is made and appropriate treatment instituted. Surgical intervention for radiation-induced bowel damage can be fraught and the opinion of an experienced surgeon should be sought if possible.

Sloan *et al.* (16) found that the degree of acute weight loss from radiotherapy was similar to the degree of weight loss induced by chemotherapy in patients who had no evidence of residual disease after operation. They also found that the effects of radiotherapy and chemotherapy were additive for those patients who received both treatments in succession.

The immediate impact of major gastrointestinal surgery has been examined in two prospective randomized studies (5, 7). Weight loss and a fall in serum albumin usually occurs, irrespective of whether or not the patient has lost weight prior to the operation. Some of the weight loss is due to the removal of the cancer, (16) along with fluid losses and catabolic effects.

Surgery may have effects on nutrition if there is disruption of deglutition either from tissue or nerve damage, persistent stricture or fistulae, or short-bowel syndrome. Gastrectomized patients can experience malnutrition if post-prandial symptoms occur. These effects can be prevented by appropriate management. (17)

INFECTION AND CACHEXIA

Chronic bacterial infection can reproduce many of the effects of advanced cancer including symptoms and signs of the anorexia–cachexia syndrome. Examples include infections associated with head and neck cancers, cavitating lung cancers, fungating tumors, and pelvic tumors associated with abscess formation. Features which suggest infection include fevers and rigors, signs of inflammation, offensive discharge, and aggravation of local pain. If the infection cannot be relieved by drainage, antibiotics which are directed against anaerobes can relieve the symptoms and reverse anorexia.

EFFECTS OF CACHEXIA ON RESPONSE TO ANTINEOPLASTIC TREATMENTS

Dewys *et al.* (4) found that weight loss was an indicator of a poorer prognosis irrespective of the diagnosis. There was also an association between weight loss and response to chemotherapy. Breast cancer patients with weight loss were less likely to respond with a complete or partial remission (44 versus 61%). A similar trend was observed for patients with acute leukemia, colon cancer, and non-small cell lung cancer but the differences were not statistically significant. No differences were noted for the other diagnosis groups. In a study which randomized patients receiving chemotherapy for testicular cancer, the trend was for lower complete remission rates in patients with significant (> 6%) weight loss. (14)

Weight loss can reduce the tolerance of patients to radiotherapy. Kinsella *et al.* (18) studied the effect of nutritional support in patients receiving pelvic radiotherapy. Patients who had lost weight and who had not received intravenous nutritional support were more likely to require unscheduled treatment breaks for radiation enteritis and were more likely to require medication to relieve gut symptoms.

Malnutrition from any cause will increase the mortality and morbidity from a major operation. (19) Two prospective randomized studies have examined the effect of pre-operative weight loss on the results of surgery for gastrointestinal malignancies. Both studies were controlled trials of perioperative parenteral nutrition in which there were three study groups comprising patients with minimal weight loss (less than 4.5 kg), patients with weight loss greater than 4.5 kg who did not receive hyperalimentation, and patients with significant weight loss who received hyperalimentation. Holter and Fischer (7) found an increased incidence of major postoperative complications (prolonged ileus, intestinal obstruction, fistula formation, wound disruption, and anastomotic leak), minor complications (pulmonary atelectasis, urinary tract infection, and wound erythema), and mortality in patients with significant weight loss.

However, Thompson *et al.* (5) did not find any significant difference in the rate of complications, major or minor.

The acute effects of surgery, radiotherapy, or chemotherapy on nutritional status are usually short-lived in patients who are rendered disease-free. However, patients with persistent or recurrent disease will manifest continued weight loss due to the disease. (16) If the disease recurs quickly and is not readily apparent, difficulties may arise when the patient is continually reassured that all should be well.

CONCLUSIONS

Cancer is commonly associated with cachexia and weight loss. Approximately half of the patients presenting for treatment will have significant weight loss, increasing to over 75% of patients who are terminally ill. The frequency of weight loss depends on the diagnosis. Other variables such as stage of disease, age, and sex are not associated with weight loss, although women are more likely to experience loss of appetite. Anticancer treatments can cause weight loss but the effects are usually short-lived if the patient achieves remission. Malnourished patients have a poorer prognosis and are less likely to respond to treatment. Aggressive nutritional support is only of proven clinical benefit in a select group of patients. When presenting for treatment, patients with lymphoma and breast cancer have a lower incidence of weight loss (less than 50%), lung, colon, and prostrate cancers have an intermediate incidence (50–60%), and gastric and pancreatic cancers produce the highest incidence (greater than 80%). In the terminal phase, breast cancer patients are still less likely to have weight loss.

REFERENCES

1. Higginson I. Epidemiologically based needs assessment for palliative and terminal care. Leeds: NHS Executive, in press.

2. Higginson I, Priest P, McCarthy M. Are bereaved family members a valid proxy for a patient's assessment of dying? Soc Sci Med 1994;38(4):553–7.
3. Bruera E, MacDonald RN. Nutrition in cancer patients: an update and review of our experience. J Pain Symptom Manage 1988;3:133–40.
4. Dewys WD, Begg C, Lavin PT et al. Prognostic effect of weight loss prior to chemotherapy in cancer patients. Am J Med 1980;69:491–6.
5. Thompson BR, Julian TB, Stremple JF. Perioperative total parenteral nutrition in patients with gastrointestinal cancer. J Surgery Res 1981;30:497–500.
6. Muller JM, Brenner U, Dienst C, Pichlmaier H. Preoperative parenteral feeding in patients with gastrointestinal carcinoma. Lancet 1982;i:68–71.
7. Holter AR, Fischer JE. The effects of perioperative hyperalimentation on complications in patients with carcinoma and weight loss. J Surgery Res 1977;23:31–4.
8. Curtis EB. Common symptoms in patients with advanced cancer. J Palliat Care 1991;7(2):25–9.
9. Dunlop GM. A study of relative frequency and importance of gastrointestinal symptoms, and weakness in patients with far advanced cancer: student paper. Palliat Med 1989;4:37–43.
10. Coyle N, Adelhardt J, Foley KM, Portenoy RK. Character of terminal illness in the advanced cancer patient: pain and other symptoms during the last four weeks. J Pain Symptom Manage 1990;5:83–93.
11. Brescia FJ, Adler D, Gray G, Ryan MA, Cimino J, Mamtani R. Hospitalized advanced cancer patients: a profile. J Pain Symptom Manage 1990;5(4):221–7.
12. Seale C, Cartwright A. The year before death. Aldershot: Avebury, 1994.
13. Mitchell EP, Schein PS. Gastrointestinal toxicity of chemotherapeutic agents. Seminars Oncol 1982;9:52–64.
14. Samuels ML, Selig DE, Ogden S et al. IV hyperalimentation and chemotherapy for stage III testicular cancer: a randomized study. Cancer Treat Rep 1981;65:615–27.
15. Valdivieso M, Bodey GP, Benjamin RS et al. Role of intravenous hyperalimentation as an adjunct to intensive chemotherapy for small cell bronchogenic carcinoma. Cancer Treat Rep 1981;65:145–50.
16. Sloan GM, Maher M, Brennan MF. Nutritional effects of surgery, radiation therapy, and adjuvant chemotherapy for soft tissue sarcomas. Am J Clin Nutr 1981;34:1094–102.
17. Lawrence W. Nutritional consequences of surgical resection of the gastrointestinal tract for cancer. Cancer Res 1977;37:2379–86.
18. Kinsella TJ, Malcolm AW, Bothe A et al. Prospective study of nutritional support during pelvic irradiation. Int J Radiat Oncol Biol Phys. 1981;7:543–8.
19. Muller JM, Keller HW, Brenner U, Holzmuller W. Indications and effects of preoperative parenteral nutrition. World J Surgery 1986;10:53–63.

6

The assessment of the nutritional status, caloric intake, and appetite of patients with advanced cancer

Rachel Burman and Joe Chamberlain

INTRODUCTION

It has been well established in other chapters that cachexia and anorexia are frequent and distressing complications of advanced cancer. This chapter reviews the alternative approaches to the assessment of nutritional status, caloric intake, and appetite, the suitability for patients with advanced cancer, and the clinical utility of these methods. Nutritional assessment of a patient with cancer may be carried out, with reference to standard values, to assess the status of the patient with regards to their disease or suitability for treatment. It may also be performed longitudinally to monitor and measure changes in response to the tumor itself, antitumor therapy, or other interventions such as parentral/enteral feeding or appetite stimulants. The assessment may be direct or by measuring a particular component of body composition. For this a four-compartment model is sometimes used (see fig. 6.1).

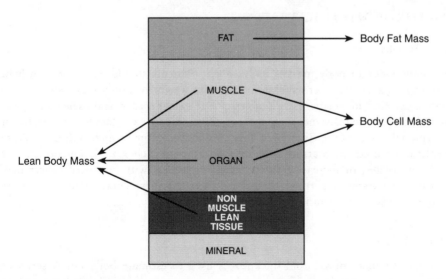

Table 6.1 Four-compartmental model of body composition.

There are many tests for nutritional assessment and the evaluation of a patient is usually by a combination of the different methods listed below:

(1) clinical assessment;

(2) anthropometric tests;

(3) dynometry;

(4) laboratory tests;

(5) infrared interactance tests;

(6) impedance/resistance tests;

(7) research methods

These are reviewed in more detail in turn.

CLINICAL ASSESSMENT

Clinical examination and observation are not to be underestimated as methods of assessing nutritional status. Work done by Baker *et al.* (1) showed agreement between multiple objective measurements and clinical assessment in the identification of 48 out of 59 patients as either normal, moderately, or severely malnourished. Specific clinical signs are associated with particular deficiencies such as pitting of the nails with iron deficiency or severe apthous ulceration with folinic acid deficiency as seen in patients undergoing chemotherapy.

ANTHROPOMETRIC TESTS

Body weight

A simple index of body mass is body weight. Patients should be weighed in light clothing on accurately zeroed scales. The body weight recorded may be compared with a pre-morbid weight or with tables of ideal weights such as those issued by the Metropolitan Life Insurance Company. (2) Percentage weight loss is an indicator of nutritional status. Often a weight loss of 10% or more, which indicates severe depletion, is used as a starting criterion for studies of cachexia. (3) The presence of oedema, ascites, or increasing tumor mass in patients with advanced cancer may distort this parameter particularly in longitudinal studies. These findings are often quoted as exclusion criteria for many trials.

Skinfold thickness

The measurement of skinfold thickness is used to estimate body fat. A series of regression equations (4) has been developed comparing body density measured by underwater weighing to multiple skinfold measurements. The total body fat is then predicted from body density. (5, 6) Skinfold thickness is measured by pinching a sample of skin and subcutaneous fat between a pair of calipers. These calipers are of standard area and deliver a standard pressure. The recognized sites for sampling are the triceps skinfold, biceps skinfold, and subscapular and suprailiac skinfolds. This method makes several assumptions, that the subcutaneous adipose tissue is a reflection of a constant proportion of total body fat and that the average thickness of adipose tissue is the same as that at the selected sites.

There are many possibilities for errors in this technique. It relies on observer expertise and there must be careful attention to accurate measurement siting if longitudinal studies are being performed. There is variability in the compressibility of adipose tissue with age and fitness. The skinfolds of patients with oedema and excess water content in their tissues will lead to an overestimate of body fat. The tables of prediction equations have usually been developed measuring a young and fit population and may not be valid in a special population such as patients with advanced cancer.

Mid-arm circumference

Measurement of the mid upper arm circumference (MUAC) in combination with the measurement of the triceps skinfold thickness (TSF) as described above can be used to estimate the mid-arm muscle circumference (MAMC):

$$\text{MAMC (cm)} = \text{MUAC (cm)} = -\Pi\text{TSF (cm)}$$

This estimate of the muscle arm circumference gives an indication of the body's muscle mass and hence its protein reserve. These measurements can be further refined by calculating cross-sectional fat (F) and muscle areas (M).

$$F = \frac{\text{RSF} \times \text{MUAC}}{2} + \frac{\Pi\text{TSF}^2}{4}$$

$$M = \frac{(\text{MUAC} - \Pi\text{TSF})^2}{4\Pi}$$

This assumes that the mid-arm is circular and the triceps skinfold is twice the average fat rim diameter. The results of these calculations do not compare unfavourably with direct measurements by computed tomography (CT) scanning. (7)

Symreng *et al.* (8) showed that in using only one of the above parameters 22% of the normal population and 88% of hospital patients would be classified as abnormal; this figure dropped to 28% of hospital patients when at least three parameters were applied. This emphasizes the need to carry out a combination of the above tests for improved accuracy.

The anthropometric tests described above have the possibility of multiple measurement errors and as has already been stated rely on progression equations which do not necessarily relate to cancer patient population. They are, however, cheap, quick, and simple tests to perform which do not require expensive equipment. The ease and speed of measurement is particularly relevant to patients suffering advanced cancer.

DYNAMOMETRY

The grip strength as measured by a dynanometer has been investigated as an index of muscle function. (9) Studies on post-operative patients (10) have shown it to be a sensitive and simply applied prognostic tool. It has been used in some studies of cancer patients. It must be remembered that the non-dominant hand is used to eliminate any previous training or repeated use of the dominant hand.

LABORATORY TESTS

Plasma protein analysis

The protein body compartment is responsible for tissue function, protein synthesis, and immune competence. The immunological tests normally carried out in nutritional assessment which look at lymphocyte activity are of no relevance in cancer patients. This is because of the effects of antineoplastic treatments and the direct immunosuppression of the disease.

Similarly measuring rapid turnover proteins such as thyroxin-binding prealbumin and retinol-binding protein is less relevant in cancer patients compared to others because of the very short half-lives: most advanced cancer patients exhibit chronic malnutrition. By the same token, these proteins are the most sensitive indicators of a change in nutritional status.

Serum albumin is a reliable indicator of visceral protein status as albumin has a half-life of 19 days (11) and is often one of the parameters measured in cancer cachexia studies. (12, 13)

Urinary metabolite excretion

Urinary creatinine and creatinine/height index

Ninety-eight per cent of creatinine is found in the form of creatinine phosphate located in skeletal muscle. Twenty-four hour collection of urine to assess creatinine excretion is used to estimate muscle mass. The creatinine height index (CHI) is defined as the urinary creatinine excretion over 24 hours expressed as a percentage of the value expected in a normal subject of the same height. It is one of the basic nutritional assessment variables often used in studies. (14) There are several factors which affect the validity of this test. Creatinine is filtered and secreted in the kidney and the patient must therefore have unimpaired renal function. There is large intraindividual variability in creatinine excretion and this needs to be reduced by patients being on restricted meat-free diets whilst undergoing investigation. Patients, their carers, or staff must also accurately time the 24 hour collection or a large margin of error is introduced. (15) To minimize these errors it is recommended that three consecutive collections are made.

3–Methyl histidine excretion (3–MH)

Research is currently evaluating 3–MH excretion as a safe non-invasive marker of muscle protein breakdown. (16)

INFRARED INTERACTANCE

This method employs the principle of light absorption. The body is irradiated with near infrared light which is reflected, absorbed, or transmitted depending on the characteristics of the tissue it hits. A computerized spectrometer with a scanning monochromator and fibre optic probe scans over a wavelength range of 700–1100 nm. The signal transmits to a depth of 1 cm. Predictive equations based on calibrated standards interpret the optical densities measured to predict total body fat. Although this is a simple non-invasive procedure it has the disadvantage of sampling regional adipose tissue deposits to predict total body fat and these samples are only 1 cm thick. (17)

BIOIMPEDANCE/RESISTANCE AND ELECTROCONDUCTIVITY

Whole-body impedance or resistance is a relatively new method of assessing body composition. It is based on the measurement of resistance of the body to the flow of an alternating electrical current. Bioelectrically resistance is a function of geometry and its electrolyte composition.

Impedance is the sum of resistance plus reactance. The reactive component of the body is so small as to be ignored. Resistance is therefore an approximation of impedance. Four self-adhesive surface electrodes are placed at the extremities on the non-dominant side of the body. A small current is passed across the body from the distal to proximal electrodes. The voltage drop across the body is measured. Resistance is then calculated using the formula

$$\text{Resistance} = \frac{voltage}{current}$$

The total body water (TBW) is estimated by this method because fat is a poor conductor compared to lean tissue which is high in conducting water and electrolyte content. The fat-free mass (FFM) can be estimated from the TBW by assuming that it is 73% water. The formula is

Body fat (BF) = total body weight - (FFM)

This is a rapid and safe bedside technique but only measures resistance at the extremities and therefore is less accurate in looking at patients whose weight loss is predominantly from their viscera or abdomen. Baumgartner *et al.* (18) have shown that as whole-body resistance is primarily in the arms and legs, body composition can be estimated accurately from just a length of arm or leg. This is better for the investigation of immobile patients. Conslick *et al.* (19) have showed little difference in the accuracy of prediction of body composition between anthropometric tests and bioimpedance.

Electroconductivity employs the principle that lean tissue conducts electrical current far better than andipose tissue. (20) The patient is placed in an electromagnetic field and the change in impedance is measured. Prediction equations have been made to estimate the lean body mass with excellent results. (20)

RESEARCH TECHNIQUES

Computed tomgraphy (CT) magnetic resonance imaging (MRI) and ultrasound imaging

All three of these techniques can directly visualize both adipose tissue and non-fat tissue in the sections of the body scanned.

CT scanning

The technique constructs a two-dimensional image of an area connecting small differences in X-ray attenuation to differences in the densities of various tissues by computer. Predictive equations have been derived to determine the total and visceral adipose tissue following serial CT measurements. (21, 22) The constraints on this method are cost and general availability in addition to the exposure to ionizing radiation. Each CT scan delivers a dose of 1.5–3.0 Gy.

Seidell *et al.* (23) have shown comparably accurate measurements between this method and anthropometric studies.

MRI scanning

Unlike CT scanning there is no exposure to ionizing radiation with this technique. It uses the principle that nuclei act as magnets and will align with an external magnetic field when it is applied across the body. The orientation of these nuclei can be altered by the application of radiofrequency waves. When this ceases the nuclei emit the radio frequency they have absorbed. These signals form the MRI image.

In this way the MRI scanner can be used to image the nuclei of carbon, nitrogen, and chlorine as well as adipose tissue. The hydrogen nucleus is the most amenable to this method and this makes studies of total body water possible. Seidell *et al.* (24) have compared CT results with those obtained with MRI scans.

Ultrasound scanning

Adipose tissue thickness has been measured by this method. Scans taken at various areas of the body can be used to estimate total adipose tissue in a similar way to skinfold thickness measurements taken with calipers.

Dual photon absorptiometry (DPA)/dual energy X-ray absorptiometry (DEXA)

Photons are generated either from a gadolinium source (DPA) or an X-ray source (DEXA). These are scanned over the patient at two different energy levels and the differential absorption of photons is measured. This technique has been used for some time to assess the bone mineral content of the spine and many institutions already have the equipment available for patients with osteoporosis. In addition, to mineral measurements it can determine the percentage of fat in non-bone tissue and, thus, the lean body mass with only the addition of the necessary software. Mazess *et al.* (25) had favorable results estimating total body composition by this method as compared to densitometry. Although Roubenoff *et al.* (26) suggested caution before this technique is used as a gold standard, it is likely to become a more widespread way of determining body composition by relatively direct analysis.

Neutron activation analysis (NAA)

This is currently the only available technique for the direct measurement of a variety of the elements of body composition. An absolute direct measurement of the amount of nitrogen, chloride, calcium, sodium, and phosphorous is possible. The individual is irradiated by a beam of fast neutrons which are caught by the target elements within the body. Unstable isotopes of these elements are created which then decay back to a stable state emitting a characteristic gamma energy which can be quantified by gamma spectograph analysis.

The ability to determine absolute total body nitrogen (TBN) values allows the estimation of the muscle and non-muscle mass. In combination with the measurement of total body calcium from which bone mineral mass can be quantified, a calculation of body fat can be made (see four-compartment model of human body composition in Fig. 6.1).

Cohn *et al.* (27, 28) have been able to assess cancer patients and assess cellular mass and lean body mass by this technique. NAA of total body nitrogen is an index of lean body mass, as potassium is almost exclusively an intracellular cation found in muscle and viscera.

Routine use of this accurate and direct method of assessment is prohibited by the cost and the need for specially trained staff. The use of ionizing radiation is less worrying in patients with advanced cancer than in younger or fitter patients.

Whole-body potassium estimation

The body naturally contains the potassium isotope ^{40}K (0.012%). This isotope emits gamma irradiation at 1.46 MeV and this can be measured *in vivo* by using a whole-body counter. Potassium is an intracellular cation which does not exist in adipose tissue. As ^{40}K represents a fixed proportion of the total body potassium it may be used to estimate the fat-free mass. (29)

Quantification of total body potassium requires specially constructed body counters with expensive shielding to exclude background irradiation. This makes it an expensive technique. Recent developments using four pi ^{40}K counting have reduced the expense and the need for the shielding. The results have been statistically good in comparison with other techniques. (30)

Total body water estimation

The estimation of total body water (TBW) uses the principle of dilution. Water occupies the fat-free mass in a fixed proportion of the lean body mass calculated as 73.2%. Fat is assumed to be anhydrous. Szeluga *et al.* (31) have shown this to be untrue as they demonstrated that adipose tissue contained 15% water by weight. Various isotopes have been used including those of hydrogen, deuterium, and tritium. The patient ingests or is injected with the isotope and the concentration excreted in the breathe, urine, or plasma water is then determined. The isotope dilution technique assumes that the isotope has the same distribution volume as water. Recently work has been done using ^{18}O as this avoids exchange of the label with non-aqueous hydrogen. (32)

ASSESSMENT OF CALORIC INTAKE

Unlike the assessment of nutritional status there are few simple and reliable methods for the assessment of food intake.

The first methods were described up to 60 years ago (33) and apart from a new method described by Bruera *et al.* (32) little has changed.

Weighed dietary records

This is theoretically most accurate as the actual weights of all the food and drink are recorded at the time of consumption. If energy-yielding nutrients only are being assessed then, in a patient with stable eating habits, 7 days should be long enough to assess caloric intake (35) with an acceptable standard error. The study should be continued for 14 days if vitamin and mineral intake are also of interest. The calorie intake can be calculated from actual weights of foodstuffs by use of food tables published in the UK by the Royal Society of Chemistry and the Ministry of Agriculture and Fisheries.

Unweighed dietary records

Patients can be asked to record food intake by estimating food quantities with reference to standard portions or household measures. This may be less demanding of the patient but it is obviously less accurate. A check of the dietary record can be made by a 24-hour collection of urinary nitrogen output.

In studies of cachexia or its potential treatments in patients with advanced cancer, caloric intake has been most often assessed by the three methods described below.

Recall methods

Caloric assessment is made by calculating the calories from a 24-hour recall dietary history taken from the patient at regular follow-up visits as in work done by Wilcox *et al.* (36) assessing the effects of prednisolone.

Bruera *et al.* (37) used a single 7-day direct recall questionnaire when looking at the association between malnutrition and calorie intake. This method was also used by Bryson *et al.* (38) when looking at caloric intake in benign and malignant gastro-intestinal disease. This may be a difficult task to ask a patient with advanced cancer to do because of the potential effect of the disease or drug treatment on memory.

Prospective records

In various studies prospective records of dietary intake and hence calories are done at set times through the follow-up of the trial (see Bruning *et al.*, (39) and work done by Bruera *et al.* (40) on methylprednisolene).

Third person percentual evaluation

Bruera *et al.* (34) described the training of nurses and volunteers in the calculation, by percentage, of how much of a foodstuff had been consumed from various receptacles. All patients' food was weighed before and after every meal and the actual caloric intake of the patient was calculated. At the same time the nurse or volunteer calculated the percentage of food taken by inspection at each meal, each foodstuff being calculated separately. A good correlation was shown between this method and the actual calories calculated. The 24-hours recall method, although more accurate, had significantly worse results than the percentual evaluation method. This method was again used successfully (3) with work done on a controlled trial of megestrol acetate. A percentual evaluation of the caloric intake was carried out using a predetermined menu on set days throughout the trial.

APPETITE ASSESSMENT

A review of the literature on studies of cachexia and its treatment in advanced cancer shows that there are two main methods used to assess appetite, if it is assessed at all.

Visual analog scale

Very poor 0 mm   100 mm Very good

The patient is asked how they would describe their appetite from very poor to very good and to represent it by a mark on the visual analog scale (see above). They are asked to perform this at various points during the trial. (12, 40)

Subjective patient questionnaire

In this method patients are asked, at various points of follow-up during a trial, a subjective questionnaire about their appetite and sense of well-being; for example, do you feel your appetite has improved since entering the trial? This technique was used in the work of Loprinzi *et al.* (13) and Kardinal *et al.* (41)

CONCLUSION

There are many ways to assess the nutritional status of a patient with advanced cancer. They range from the rapid, simple, and inexpensive to research methods which require highly trained staff and expensive equipment. Assessment of appetite and caloric intake is less well researched and established. Collaboration with our dietetic colleagues, together with the further development of the new research methods with a more reliable direct assessment of nutritional status will facilitate research protocols. Treatments of cachexia may then be more easily investigated and validated. This distressing and debilitating symptom of advanced cancer may then become less common.

REFERENCES

1. Baker JP, Detsky AS, Wesson DE. A comparison of clinical judgement and objective measurements. New Eng Med 1982; 306: 969–88.
2. Metropolitan Life Insurance Company Statistical Bulletin 1983; 64: 1–9.
3. Bruera E, Macmillan KA. A controlled trial of Megestrol Acetate on appetite, caloric intake, nutritional status and other symptoms in patients with advanced cancer. Cancer 1990; 66: 1279–82.
4. Durnin JVGA, Womersley J. Body fat assessed from total body density and its estimation from skinfold thickness: measurements on 481 men and women from 16 to 72 yrs. Br Nutr 1973; 32: 77–97.
5. Lohman TG. Skinfolds and body density and their relation to body fatness: a review. Human Biol 1981; 53: 181–225.
6. Durnin JVGA, Satwani KMJ. Variations in the assessment of the fat content of the human body due to experimental technique in measuring body density. Ann Human Biol 1982; 9: 221–5.
7. Heymsfield SB. Anthropometric measurement of muscle mass: revised equations for calculating bone free arm muscle area. Am J Clin Nutr 1982;36:680–90.
8. Symreng T, Anderberg B. Nutritional assessment and clinical course in 112 elective surgical patients. Acta Chir Scand 1983; 149: 657–62.
9. Griffin CDM, Clark RG. A comparison of the Sheffield prognostic index with forearm muscle dynamometry in patients from Sheffield undergoing major abdominal and urological surgery. Clin Nutr 1984; 3:147–51.
10. Hunt DR, Rowlands BJ, Johnston D. Handgrip strength: a simple prognostic indicator in surgical patients. J Parent Ent Nutr 1985; 701–4.
11. Starker PM, Gump FE, Askanazi J. Serum albumin levels as an index of nutritional support. Surgery 1982; 195–9.
12. Downer S, Joel S. A double blind placebo controlled trial of medroxyprogesterone acetate in cancer cachexia. Br J Cancer 1993; 67: 1102–5.
13. Loprinski CL, Michalak JC, Schaid DL. Phase three evaluation of four doses of Megestrol Acetate as therapy for patients with cancer anorexia or cachexia. J Clin Oncol 1993; 11: 762–7.
14. Tchekmedyian NS, Tait N, Moody M.. Appetite stimulation with Megestrol Acetate in cachetic cancer patients. Seminar Oncol 1986; 4: 37–43.
15. Forbes GB, Bruning GJ. Urinary creatinine excretion and lean body mass. Am J Clin Nutr 1976; 29: 1359–66.
16. Long CL, Haverburg, Young VR. Metabolism of 3-methylhistidine in man. Metabolism 1975; 24: 929–35.
17. Lukaski HC. Methods of assessment of human body composition traditional and new. Am Soc Clin Nutr 1987; 46: 537–56.
18. Baumgartner RN, Chumlea WC, Roche AF. Estimation of body composition from bioelectric impedance of body segments. Am J Clin Nutr 1989; 50: 221–6.
19. Conlisk EA, Haas JD, Martinez EJ et al. Predicting body composition from anthropometry and bioimpedance. Am J Clin Nutr 1992; 55: 1051–9.
20. Presta E, Wang J, Harrison CG et al. Measurement of total body electrical conductivity a new method for estimating body composition. Am J Clin Nutr 1983; 37:735–9.
21. Kvist H, Chowdhury B, Sjostrom L. Adipose tissue volume determination in males by computed tomography. Int J Obesity 1988; 12: 249–66.
22. Kvist H, Chowdhury B, Grangard U et al. Predictive equations of total and visceral adipose tissue volumes derived from measurements with C-T scanning in adult men and women. Am J Clin Nutr 1988; 48: 1351–61.
23. Seidell JC, Oosterlee A, Thijssen MAO et al. Assessment of intra-abdominal fat relation between anthropometry and C-T scanning. Am J Clin Nutr 1987; 45: 7–13.

24. Seidell JC, Bakker CJG, van der Kooy K. Imaging techniques for measuring adipose tissue distribution a comparison between CT and 1.5-T magnetic resonance. Am Soc Clin Nutr 1990; 51:953–7.

25. Mazess RB, Barden HS, Bisek JP et al. Dual energy X-ray absorptionmetry for total body and regional bone mineral and soft tissue composition. Am J Clin Nutr 1990; 51: 1106–12.

26. Roubenoff R, Kehayias JJ, Dawson-Hughes B et al. Use of dual energy X ray absorptiometry in composition studies; not yet a gold standard. Am J Clin Nutr 1993; 58: 589–91.

27. Cohn SH, Ellis KJ, Vartsky D et al. Comparison of methods of estimating body fat in normal subjects and cancer patients. Am J Nutr 1981; 34: 2839–47.

28. Cohn SH et al. Assessment of cellular mass and lean body mass by noninvasive techniques. J Lab Clin Med 1985; 105: 305–11.

29. Garrow JS et al. New approaches to body composition. Am J Clin Nutr 1982; 35: 1152–7.

30. Pierson NJ Jr, Wang J, Thorton JC. Body potassium by four pi-K counting; an anthropometric correction. Am J Physiol 1984; 246: F234–9.

31. Szeluga DJ et al. Nutritional assessment by isotope dilution analysis of body composition. Am J Clin Nutr 1984; 40: 847–54.

32. Schoeller DA, van Santer E, Peterson DW et al. Total body water measurement in humans with 18-O and 2H water. Am J Clin Nutr 1980; 33: 2686–93.

33. Widdowson EM. A study of English diets by an individual method. Part One men. J Hygiene 1936; 36: 269–92.

34. Bruera E, Chadwicks S, Cowan L et al. Caloric intake assessment in advanced cancer patients: a comparison of three methods. Cancer Treat Rep 1986; 70: 981–3.

35. Bingham J. The dietary assessment of individuals; methods accuracy, new techniques and recommendations. Nutr Abstr Rev 1987; 57: 705–42.

36. Willcox J, Corr J, Shaw J et al. Prednisolone as an appetite stimulant in patients with cancer. BMJ 1984; 288: 27.

37. Bruera E, Carrara S, Roca E et al. Association between malnutrition and caloric intake, emesis, psychological depression, glucose taste and tumour mass. Cancer Treat Rep 1984; 6873–5.

38. Bryson E, Kark A. Dietary intakes, resting metabolic rates and body nutrition in benign and malignant gastrointestinal disease. BMJ 1980; 280: 211–15.

39. Bruning P. Dietary intake, nutritional status and the wellbeing of cancer patients. Eur J Cancer Clin Oncol 21; 1449–59.

40. Bruera E, Roca E, Cedaro L et al. Action of oral methylprednisolone in terminal cancer patients; a prospective randomised double blind study. Cander Treat Rep 1985; 69: 751–54.

41. Kardinal KG, Loprinzi C, Schaid DJ et al. A controlled trial of cyproheptadine in cancer patients with anorexia-cachexia. Cancer 1990; 65: 2657–62.

7

Indications and ethical considerations in the hydration of patients with advanced cancer

Neil MacDonald and Robin Fainsinger

They gave Him wine mixed with gall — He tasted but refused to drink.

Matthew 27–34

They put a sponge soaked in vinegar on a hyssop stick — and held it to his mouth.
After he had taken the vinegar — He said, 'It is accomplished' and gave up the ghost.

John 19–29, 30

While the quotes heading this chapter are from the Bible, the tenets of most cultures and religions hold that offering food and drink to the dying are both humane and essential facets of community life. Recently, this view has been challenged on medical (the thesis that hydration may actually harm the dying), economic, and ethical grounds. The three realms are not separate as ethical or economic arguments are based on one's understanding of the biologic features of supplementary nutrition and hydration. Weiss (1) states, 'Public policy positions taken by policy actors are the result of three sets of forces: their ideologies, their interest (for example, power, reputation, financial reward), and the information they have.' Information may be selectively used to buttress ethical views. 'Better to make your case in public with scientific facts (hard) rather than soft principles (soft).' (2)

In this chapter we will consider pathophysiologic issues related to hydration. These are covered for nutrition in Chapter 6. We use our interpretation of relevant biology to buttress our view that two-dimensional ethical considerations leading one to either withhold dogmatically or maintain hydration are inappropriate and that a centre view based on patient–family wishes and the careful analysis of benefits accruing from hydration in relieving suffering must be the determinant factor.

ETHICAL CONSIDERATIONS

In their published *Guidelines on the termination of life sustaining treatment and the care of the dying*, (3) the Hastings Center outlines ethical guidelines on hydration procedures. These guidelines recognize that offering fluids to the dying has con-notations beyond biology. Nevertheless, they also clearly state that any techniques which involve the insertion of tubes, catheters, or needles into the patient's body, must be regarded as medical interventions which may be ethically terminated in certain situations. Considering the social and symbolic aspects of hydration, they also stress that the evaluation of the need for it requires both an assessment of physiological and psychological need. The Hastings group recognizes that each patient situation is different and must be carefully assessed independent of the application of rigid policies on hydration.

In their generally balanced account, a number of statements are made which are debatable. The Hastings group state that 'malnutrition and dehydration are conditions determined by chemical tests'. Furthermore, they state that the dehydrated patients may have their thirst relieved simply by moistening the lips and mouth. As will be discussed later in this chapter, because of alterations in other aspects of patient metabolism, simple chemical tests for dehydration which apply to otherwise healthy individuals can often not be relied upon in patients with advanced cancer or AIDS. Moreover, thirst is a complex symptom. Thirst is relieved immediately after drinking, long before fluid is absorbed from the gastrointestinal tract with the consequent adjustment of blood volume and osmolality. Witness the immediate gratifying resolution of thirst when we take a cold drink on a hot day. Therefore, the sensation of thirst must be influenced by receptors in the mouth and nasopharynx. Thus, it is not necessary to correct fully the stimulation of osmoreceptors in the brain, the usual mechanism inducing the sensation of thirst in dehydrated patients. Certainly, an unpleasant sensation arising from dryness of the mucous membranes of the mouth can be relieved by local application of fluid. It is not clear, however, how much fluid ingestion, reaching what area of the upper gastrointestinal tract, is required to alleviate centrally mediated thirst.

Nevertheless, these guidelines emphasizing flexibility and the use of time-limited trials to determine whether a medical intervention is indeed assisting the patient, provide a reasoned discussion on ethical aspects of hydrating patients with far-advanced illness.

While issued from a secular perspective the Hastings Center guidelines are consonant with Christian ethical views, at least as reflected in the teachings of Catholic theology. (4) The weight of Catholic church teachings over centuries clearly supports the view that 'Even natural means, such as of food and drink, can become optional if taking them requires great effort or if the hope of beneficial results (spes salutis) is not present'. (5) The quotes from The Passion Gospels which head this chapter may be symbolically relevant. In one account, Christ accepted wine and gall (which some believe contained an opiate or some other natural analgesic). In another, Christ refused fluid and shortly thereafter died.

As is common in ethical commentaries, the Hastings Center guidelines stress that patient permission must be obtained for any medical intervention and, if the patient is mentally incompetent, that family surrogates should fully understand the proposed medical intervention and provide authorization. This point is particularly important in the context of hydration, as dehydration itself serves as one of the principal direct and indirect (through its impact on drug clearance) causes of deteriorating cognitive function. It raises an interesting ethical dilemma, as the failure to recognize and appropriately treat dehydration may lead to a situation whereby the patient's wishes cannot be determined and medical attendants must fall back upon discussion with surrogates.

The argument that the decision on hydration should be made by the patient, where possible, is supported by the report from the Hastings Center (6) that states: 'a competent adult is the one individual best able to know what he or she wants and therefore has the right to decide what is in his or her own best interest'. Caregivers, however, need to keep in mind that patients can be swayed in their decisions by the manner in which information is presented to them. This is well illustrated by a recently completed study in which two palliative care units, one in Edmonton and one in Ottawa, Canada, carried out a hydration study. It is the common practice to offer parenteral hydration to patients in Edmonton and discourage parenteral hydration in Ottawa. Patients approached for consent to participate in this study on both sites appeared to have had no problem agreeing with the need for parenteral hydration in Edmonton and agreeing to the absence of parenteral hydration in Ottawa (unpublished data). This would appear to provide strong evidence of the ability of care givers to bias patients in their decision-making.

In both the United States and Canada, in an effort to maintain and improve health care at a lower cost, 'case management', 'managed care', and similar programmes are now in vogue. A core idea in these programmes is the concept of the care plan — a plan which provides guidelines for patient care in a variety of circumstances. This approach is meritorious for many reasons, not the least of which arises from the emphasis on anticipation of problems and efficient use of resources. From an ethical standpoint, care must be taken that the creation of care plans for managing the last weeks of life for patients with advanced cancer or AIDS does not lead to the over-rigid application of a hydration plan which may not be appropriate for a particular patient.

Ethical considerations of medical interventions must consider not only the patient, but family members. Depending upon the health system in their country, families will bear the cost of hydration therapy on either an in-patient or an out-patient basis. In Canada, while in-patient costs will be covered, home hydration may cost family members in the range of $75–150 a week. Aside from the economic costs, an increased burden for providing care is present for family members looking after a loved one at home. Family members may also be concerned about what they may interpret as the prolongation of a life of needless suffering. They will also be dismayed if their loved one is confused and agitated.

For most advanced cancer patients, it is debatable that hydration, by itself, prolongs life to any substantial degree (although not the focus of this chapter, hydration may prolong existence in brain-damaged patients in a persistent vegetative state). The use of subcutaneous infusion techniques for hydration simplifies the process and reduces costs but, nevertheless, hydration is associated with financial expense. If this expense is balanced by reduction of other costs which may be associated with a reduced need to treat symptoms caused by dehydration, an ethical dilemma does not arise. The possibility that hydration can cut down on agitated delirium and the associated terrible emotional cost for family members is discussed later in this chapter.

A review of other ethical guidelines published by authoritative professional bodies generally supports the acceptability of withdrawing nutrition and hydration. The situations where this is allowed hinge on three principal circumstances.

1. *Futility of therapy.* Where all parties concur that no meaningful improvement in the patient's condition will be achieved.

2. *Beneficence of therapy.* Where the patient's degree of comfort will not be improved and no benefit is achieved.

3. *Avoidance of harm.* Where providing food and fluids could actually harm the patient.

A review of recent ethical literature interpreting these circumstances provides evidence that ethical stances relate to one's interpretation of biological as well as moral principles. Ethical guidelines may reflect the author's understanding that parenteral hydration translates into the use of intravenous lines with consequent technical limitations. However, the ideal procedure for parenteral hydration involves the placement of a needle in the subcutaneous tissue, usually of the upper chest wall and the infusion of electrolyte solutions through this readily established and replaceable site (v.i.).

This technique is not burdensome, nor, unlike intravenous line placements, a potential added source of pain or patient distress. Consequently, the assessment of the balance of harmful and beneficial effects of intervention is skewed towards intervention.

Parenteral hydration may have other detrimental biological effects which influence this equation. Increased passage of urine will certainly occur, while it is postulated that more fluid may translate into more peripheral oedema and a greater risk of vomiting and accumulation of lung secretions. These concerns will be addressed later in the chapter.

It is helpful for a hospital or home-care group to formally discuss their policies on hydration, and to publish the outcome of these discussions. Modeled on guidelines on enteral feeding published by the Bioethics Centre of the University of Alberta, (7) the following guidelines for hydration may be considered.

Patient choice

1. Competent patients can accept or refuse hydration when given pertinent information.

2. For incompetent patients, a balancing of advantages and disadvantages should be undertaken. The patient's interests are paramount in decisions. Incompetent patients may be represented by a legal guardian or health care agent.

Decision-making process

1. Patients, families and friends, and caregivers should know that hydration can be ethically withheld and withdrawn.

2. Hydration should usually be initiated on a time-limited basis to allow an assessment of the advantages and disadvantages.

3. A time-limited trial of hydration is always recommended if there is doubt about the advantages or disadvantages of hydration.

4. After a decision has been made to initiate or stop hydration, the emotional impact of the decision on care givers, family members, and others must be recognized and responded to.

5. The advantages and disadvantages of hydration for family members, close friends,

care givers, and society may influence the decisions made by competent patients or made for incompetent patients.

Unless there is a contraindication, patients receiving pharmacologic agents should also receive hydration in order to limit the risk of delirium or other adverse drug effects.

As hydration is readily carried out via the subcutaneous route, cultural and emotional factors influencing the decision to use hydration can be readily accommodated without patient distress.

VOLUME DEPLETION

Hydration for treatment of volume-depleted patients is seemingly a straightforward proposition, but volume depletion is often masked in palliative care patients. The word 'dehydration' is sometimes used to encompass all volume-depletion syndromes. To avoid confusion, the term 'dehydration' should be used to describe 'relatively pure water depletion leading to hypernatremia'. (8) This situation is uncommon in palliative care. More frequently, depletions of both sodium and water are present.

A reduction in extracellular fluid volume, whatever the cause, will result in reduced skin turgor (skin elasticity), dry mucous membranes, and reduced sweating. The associated drop in circulating blood volume may cause tachycardia, postural hypotension, and oliguria. Clinically, the patient is weak, may complain of thirst, constipation, dysphagia, and trouble concentrating. The family may note confusion.

However, a normovolaemic patient with advanced cancer or AIDS may have all of these signs and symptoms. Cancer patients commonly have autonomic neuropathies, (9) which can cause changes in cardiac reflexes and could interfere with bowel function. Skin turgor is difficult to categorize in the aged or in those with the cachexia–anorexia syndrome. The sensation of thirst, secondary to increased blood osmolality or decreased blood volume may be confused with the need for water to relieve parched oral mucosa in a mouth-breathing patient or one on anticholinergic drugs. Confusion is commonly noted in many patients with advanced cancer and AIDS. (10)

Plasma protein levels and the haematocrit will increase in volume-concentrated patients, but both indices are often abnormally low in patients with advanced cancer or AIDS. Therefore, they are not helpful unless a sequence of values is available. The BUN and creatinine normally increase following the drop in renal plasma flow and glomerular filtration occurring with volume depletion. Even in the absence of renal disease, the baseline creatinine may be low in advanced cancer and AIDS patients because many of them are wasted and have lost muscle protein stores.

Although it is sometimes difficult to identify a volume-depleted state, the physician must ultimately depend on clinical judgement as laboratory techniques for assessing blood volumes remain expensive and not readily adaptable to a palliative care setting. (11)

The serum sodium *may* not convey accurate information about the total body sodium content in volume-depleted states (v.i.). For example, a drop in blood volume may trigger non-osmotic release of antidiuretic hormone (ADH) with a consequent drop in sodium values. Plasma and urine osmolality levels are variably helpful; one example: they may demonstrate that a 'pseudo-hyponatremia' secondary to plasma increase in glucose or other osmotically active substances (12) is present. Volume depleted patients may

(1) lose water in excess of sodium (hypernatremic fluid loss);

(2) lose water and sodium equally (normonatremic fluid loss);

(3) lose sodium in excess of water (hyponatremic fluid loss).

HYPERNATREMIC FLUID LOSS

A high serum sodium provides prima facie evidence for relative water depletion. A high serum sodium is unusual in palliative care patients. It occurs most frequently in patients with severe dehydration who are losing hypotonic body fluids but who cannot respond appropriately by drinking water because they are obtunded (a common feature in hypernatremic patients) and/or have a diminished sense of thirst. Clinical situations where this occurs include

(1) diabetes insipidus;

(2) fever and excess sweating;

(3) osmotic diuresis (examples include diabetes mellitus or diuresis induced by augmented urea excretion secondary to increased protein intake in patients receiving enteral and parenteral feedings) — here the urine contains an excess of non-electrolytes so that more water than electrolyte is lost;

(4) increased insensible losses following increase in ambient temperature;

(5) confused states with lack of thirst.

NORMONATREMIC VOLUME DEPLETION

This normally occurs when sodium and fluid loss are balanced. However, patients with advanced cancer often have a baseline hyponatremia prior to the onset of dehydration (v.i.). Therefore, a normal serium sodium could mask volume depletion due to primary water loss. This situation is only readily determined if prior sodium (and hacmatocrit) determinations are available.

HYPONATREMIC VOLUME DEPLETION

Hyponatraemia is commonly observed in patients with AIDS, cancer, and other chronic illnesses. (13) On occasion, the drugs patients must take may contribute to their hyponatremia. A variety of sedatives, antipsychotic drugs, and opiates may all interfere with water clearance by the kidney. Some patients, notably those with small cell carcinomas of the lung (and occasionally other tumor types), have readily identifiable causes for this finding, as their tumors inappropriately produce antidiuretic hormone. (14) Patients with inappropriate ADH secretation are presumably not hypovolemic. Some tumors, notably small cell lung cancers, may also produce or stimulate production of atrial naturetic peptide. (15) The extent of the problem and the resultant volume change in patients is, as yet, poorly characterized. In other hyponatremic patients with AIDS or cancer, a true increase in body water is not necessarily present.

The presence of hyponatremia in a patient with clinical volume depletion is not unusual. Patients may be hyponatremic, yet volume depleted, if they lose sodium in excess of water or if they have a baseline hyponatremia and sustain a balanced fluid–electrolyte loss. In hospital practices diuretics are a common cause of this condition. Many cancer patients have sequestrated fluid accumulation states, ascites may be present, or lower limb oedema secondary to partial lymphatic obstruction, severe hypoalbuminemia and anemia, or a mixture of causes. Attempts to alleviate these problems with diuretics are sometimes made and, if not carefully monitored, can accelerate hyponatremic volume depletion.

The elderly ill patient is particularly at risk of developing a volume depletion state, often with hyponatremia. Older healthy subjects usually have a disproportionate increase in body fat and a corresponding lower proportion of body water in comparison to younger adults. (16) They often have a decreased thirst reflex, (17) and altered renal responses to changes in electrolyte fluid shifts. (18)

Table 7.1   Risk factors for dehydration in the elderly

Unable to eat or drink without assistance
Enteral support without added free water
Depression
Loss of interest in self-care
Loss of memory, communication skills
Apraxia
Multiple chronic diseases
Acute infection
Polyuria related to diabetes insipidus or poorly controlled diabetes mellitus
Vomiting or diarrhea
Use of medications such as diuretics, laxatives, and sedatives
Neglect
Insensibility to thirst
Physiological renal changes

Reprinted with permission from ref. (17)

Therefore, stresses including vomiting, diarrhea and decreases in salt or water intake can readily result in a state of hyponatremic volume depletion.

Other recognized causes of hypovolemia and hyponatremia include fistulas, excess sweating, chronic renal disease, or, less commonly, Addison's disease.

Hyponatremia in advanced cancer and AIDS patients is sometimes encountered in the absence of an assignable cause. A reset osmostat has been postulated to account for some of these inexplicable cases of hyponatremia with volume depletion. Why this should occur in cancer patients is not known, although some investigators have suggested that cancer may induce changes in cell membranes through which a variety of osmotically significant organic solutes, normally confined within a cell, may be released into the extracellular fluid (ECF), resulting in a state of intracellular hypo-osmolatity and an exchange with ECF sodium needed to maintain osmotic balance. (18–20) As this process continues and as these intracellular components are exercised or metabolized, hyponatraemia will occur. Depending on fluid intake, patients may or may not be hypovolaemic.

A loss of intracellular solute and water is commonly noted in patients with weight loss and chronic wasting disorders. (21) The loss of organic solute affects the hypothalamic cells which comprise the body's 'osmostat'. They will reset their function to stimulate release of ADH at osmotic (and perhaps, volume) levels which maintain serum osmolality and serum sodium at subnormal values. Thus, the normal' baseline shifts to a serum sodium of 125–137.

Acute hyponatraemic states are associated with severe and potentially fatal alterations in brain function. In order to maintain osmotic balance between the extracellular and intracellular compartments, brain cells take on water and this consequent swelling can initially cause lethargy and mild cognitive impairment, followed, in severely affected patients, by stupor, coma, and death secondary to cerebral oedema.

Do the chronic hyponatremic states also contribute to the host of symptoms afflicting cancer patients? Certainly, lethargy, depression, and cognitive changes commonly afflict advanced cancer patients. To the author's knowledge, studies comparing the type, frequency, and severity of symptoms in hyponatremic (< 130 mEq Na) and normonatraemic cancer patients have not been carried out.

However, derivative evidence is available which suggests these possibilities:

1. In healthy subjects, the gradual development of hyponatremia following salt restriction and increased water intake caused a variety of symptoms, including apathy, exhaustion, and muscle cramps. (22) However, this model may simply represent semi-acute hyponatraemia'.

2. The psychiatric literature contains references to patients with chronic hypona-traemia whose symptoms relate to the severity of hyponatraemia and may improve following correction of the dysfunction. (23, 24) However, the causes of hyponatraemia in these cases may have little relationship to the hyponatraemia present in cancer or AIDS patients.

THE MANAGEMENT OF VOLUME DEPLETION

The controversy

The treatment of volume depletion in terminally ill patients is a very controversial topic, with numerous reports in the literature illustrating opposing points of view. The arguments for and against rehydration (25–34) can be summarized as follows:

Arguments against
1. Comatose patients do not experience pain, thirst, etc.

2. Fluid may prolong the dying process.

3. Less urine output means less need for bed pan, urinal, commode, or catheter.

4. Less gastrointestinal fluid and less vomiting.

5. Less pulmonary secretions and less cough, choking, and congestion.

6. Minimize oedema and ascites.

7. Decreased fluids and electrolyte imbalance act as natural anaesthetic for the central nervous system with decreased levels of consciousness and decreased suffering.

Arguments for

1. Dying patients are more comfortable if they receive adequate hydration.

2. There is no evidence that fluids alone prolong life to any meaningful degree.

3. Dehydration and electrolyte imbalance can cause confusion, restlessness, and neuromuscular irritability.

4. Water is administered to dying people who complain of thirst, so why not give parenteral hydration.

5. Arguments regarding poor quality of life detract from efforts to find ways to improve comfort and life quality.

6. Parenteral hydration is the minimum standard of care and discontinuing this treatment is to break a bond with the patient.

7. Withholding fluid to dying patients is the thin edge of the wedge to withholding therapies to other compromised patient groups.

The arguments for the maintenance of hydration in terminally ill patients have tended to come from 'the traditional medical model'. (26, 27, 34) A recent analysis of the use of the intravenous fluids in patients dying from a malignant disease in a tertiary care teaching hospital (37) showed that 73 out of 106 patients died with an intravenous line running. The need to hydrate terminally ill patients has been vigorously challenged, mainly by palliative care doctors and nurses (38) who have noted many terminally ill patients dying comfortably without parenteral hydration.

It would appear from these reports that many care givers have reacted to the injudicious use of intravenous fluids in dying patients and the negative effects noted from this management, by developing a policy that if intravenous fluids can cause harm in some patients, therefore giving no parenteral fluids to any dying patients is the ideal management approach.

A review of the literature indicates that most of the arguments are based on anecdotal reports that have not been substantiated with any scientific data. The anecdotal nature of the opposing points of view is well illustrated by two recent reports. (37, 38) Andrews *et al.* (37) reported on three patients managed without parenteral hydration who, it is argued, demonstrate the palliative benefits of dehydration (decreased problems of oedema, respiratory secretions and congestion, and fluid overload). In contrast, Yan and Bruera (38) reported on three terminally ill patients in whom hydration was deemed crucial in maintaining or recovering cognitive function in two patients, and in assisting in recovery and eventual discharge in a third patient.

The much repeated argument that the main symptom of dehydration is a dry mouth, which can be satisfactorily relieved by small amounts of water, ice chips, and/ or good mouth care, (29, 36, 37, 39) was considered in an article that provides the first quantitative estimate of the experience of dehydration symptoms in advanced cancer patients. (40) Consent was obtained from 52 patients who participated in a cross-sectional survey to determine the severity and distribution of the symptoms of thirst, dry mouth, bad taste, nausea, pleasure in drinking, fatigue and pain, and the association of these symptoms with objective measures of dehydration. While all symptoms with the exception of pain and nausea, appeared to be moderately severe, there was no demonstrable association between severity and fluid intake. The study did not provide evidence to support the rationale for basing the decision to begin assisted fluids on the history of fluid intake and laboratory measures if the aim is reducing thirst. The conclusions are limited by the short duration of the study. In addition, patients excluded by the study design appeared to be sicker, had significantly less fluid intake, and more aggressive mouth care. In addition, as oral fluids have been found to decrease significantly in dehydrated patients, (41) it could be argued that maintaining normal hydration in terminally ill patients can only assist in minimizing difficulties with mouth care in terminally ill patients.

The argument against hydration is summarized in a recent article that states 'Based on ... a review of the literature, it is likely that prolonged dehydration and starvation induce no pain and only limited discomfort from a dry mouth, which can be controlled. For individuals carrying an intolerable burden of illness and disability, or those who have no hope of ever again enjoying meaningful human interaction, the withdrawal of food and fluid may be considered without concern that it will add to the misery.' (42)

We would argue that a generalized statement that dehydration in dying patients is not a cause of symptom distress overlooks a few important points. (43–45)

1. Dehydration is known to cause confusion and restlessness in patients with non-terminal disease, (8, 47, 48) symptoms that are often reported in terminally ill patients (49, 50) and could be aggravated by dehydration.

2. The decreased intravascular volume and glomerular filtration rate from dehydration can result in renal failure. The accumulation of opiate metabolites in the presence of renal failure, resulting in confusion, myoclonus, and seizures, has been well documented. (54–59)

3. Dehydration has been associated with increased risk of bed sores (60) and constipation, (61, 62) particularly in geriatric patients.

It makes little sense that a patient receive drugs for agitated delirium, myoclonus, and seizures if these problems could have been prevented by the treatment of dehydration. All these problems have been frequently reported in patients in the last days of life. (36, 49, 63–65) While many terminally ill patients may die peacefully without parenteral fluids, there is some consensus on the necessity of individualizing management. (45, 66) This implies that, rather than a universal policy of hydration for all or no hydration of all, there is a need to keep in mind that the patient with agitated delirium may have dehydration as the underlying cause, while for the many terminally ill patients on medication, whose effects are mediated by renal excretion, renal failure due to dehydration is not necessarily a benign complication.

HYPODERMOCLYSIS

The term hypodermoclysis (HDC) was initially used to describe the infusion of fluids into the subcutaneous space. (68) However, HDC has been used not only as a method of fluid replacement, but has also become popular as a method for delivery of symptom control. (69–71) It is worth nothing that many articles criticizing the use of parenteral hydration in terminally ill patients refer only to parenteral hydration by the intravenous route. (26, 33, 36, 72)

HDC, although widely used in clinical practice in the 1940s and 1950s, was largely replaced by intravenous infusion and is rarely used today, with many physicians being unfamiliar and unexposed to this technique. There have recently been a number of articles discussing HDC and the potential advantages over intravenous therapy. (38, 43, 44, 70, 71, 73) Despite this, a recent article on physician attitudes in the management of dehydration in dying patients (74) did not offer HDC as a means of parenteral hydration in a terminally ill patient.

The safety of HDC has been well documented, with numerous reports testifying to its usefulness and low incidence of adverse effects. Schen and Singer-Edelstein (75) reported HDC as being an exceptionally safe and occasionally life-saving means of fluid replacement. In their experience, in four out of 270 patients the only significant problem reported was local oedema. A follow-up report (76) noted that in nine out of 634 patients the most common side-effect was overloading, causing either oedema or heart failure. One patient developed local infection, with two patients developing ecchymosis. The authors suggested avoiding HDC in patients with blood coagulation disorders, giving fluid slowly if the patient had a pre-existing heart disorder, and constantly checking for oedema.

Hays (70) supported HDC as an adequate method of symptom control for terminal cancer patients. During a 3-year period only one patient developed cellulitis, and two patients had allergic reactions, with hives and erythema in the subcutaneous site. Bruera *et al*. (69) reported that in 58 treated patients, the side-effects were local infection in two cases and bruising in another two.

Fainsinger *et al*. (44) reported a prospective open study of 100 consecutive patients dying on a palliative care unit. Sixty-nine out of 100 patients received HDC for an average of 14 + 18 days during an average admission of 35 + 41 days. The HDC was well tolerated in most patients who were given an average volume of 1203 + 505 ml per day. Problems noted that led to discontinuation of HDC were pulmonary oedema in one patient, generalized oedema in three patients, and local allergic reactions to hyaluronidase in two patients. The average subcutaneous site duration was 4.7 + 5.4 days. The most common reasons for site change were poor absorption (47%), inflammation (37%), and bleeding or bruising (11%).

Hyaluronidase is an enzyme that breaks down hyaluronic acid and thus apparently aids the rapid diffusion and absorption of injected fluids by temporarily lysing the normal interstitial barrier, which mainly consists of hyaluronic acid. (73, 77) The amount of hyaluronidase recommended varies from 150 to 750 units per litre. (43, 69–71, 73) The ideal amount of hyaluronidase requires further scientific study and at present remains controversial. (78, 79) Our most recent experience has been that 750 units of hyaluronidase is unnecessary in most patients and our common practice of using 150 units of hyaluronidase in each litre has been successful in the majority of patients.

Most reports (69–71, 73, 75–77, 80, 81) recommended the use of solutions with electrolytes such as normal saline or two-thirds 5% dextrose and one-third saline, since non-electrolyte solutions have been reported to draw fluid into the interstitial space. Rates of infusion ranging from 20 to 120 ml per hour are quoted as being well tolerated in most patients. However, this is also controversial, with single cases (73) and small studies (82) reporting patients tolerating boluses of up to 500 ml per hour. We are presently conducting a study assessing the tolerance of patients to boluses of 500 cc over 1 hour two or three times per day. One hundred and fifty units of hyaluronidase is given to the subcutaneous site prior to the bolus infusion. Initial results indicate that this is well tolerated in the majority of patients.

HDC offers many advantages over the intravenous route. (43, 73)

1. Intravenous access can be difficult in patients with advanced disease.

2. HDC can be started by any staff member able to give a subcutaneous injection, without the need for a physician or IV team.

3. HDC can be stopped and started without concern for thrombosis in the subcutaneous needle.

4. Hospitalization can be avoided or shortened in some patients.

5. Subcutaneous HDC sites often last for several days.

HDC clearly offers a more convenient way of maintaining hydration in patients with advanced disease, with patients being individually assessed for tolerance to varying rates of infusion and requirements of hyaluronidase.

CONCLUSION

As has been pointed out, (83) the core of the dehydration debate does not lie with the choice of the most effective symptom control technique. The main problem remains the decision as to whether to supply a patient unable to sustain an adequate oral intake of fluids with parenterally administered hydration. It is clear from a review of the literature that the mainly anecdotal data reported to date are insufficient to reach a final conclusion. We would argue, however, that there is sufficient information available to cast some doubt on the belief that dehydration in the terminally ill is beneficial for all dying patients. It is hoped that further scientific research in the future will provide more definitive answers. In the meantime, it would seem prudent

(The authors thank Dr Mortimer Levy, Director of the Division of Nephrology, Royal Victoria, Montreal, for revviewing the chapter and assisting the authors with the chapter's outline of physiologic principles.)

to follow a compromise approach as follows: while some dying patients may not suffer any ill effects from dehydration, there might be others who do manifest symptoms, such as confusion or opiate toxicity, whose symptoms could well be alleviated by parenteral hydration.

REFERENCES

1. Weiss CH. Ideology, interests, and information. In: Callahan D, Jennings B (eds.) In ethics, the social sciences and policy analysis. New York: Plenum Press, c1983: p. 221.
2. Callahan D. Medical futility, medical necessity — the problem without a name. P-35. Hastings Center Rep 1991; 21(4) 30–35.
3. Hastings Center. Guidelines on the termination of life-sustaining treatment and the care of the dying. Indiana University Press, 1987. Briarcliff Manor, NY: The Center, c1987.
4. Paris JJ, McCormick RA. The Catholic tradition on the use of nutrition and fluids. Am 1987; 2 May: 356–62.
5. Cronin DA. The moral law in regard to the ordinary and extraordinary means of preserving life (dissertation). Gregorian University.
6. Green W. Setting boundaries for artificial feeding. Hastings Center Rep. 1984; December 9–13, 14(6): 8–10.
7. Interdisciplinary Committee on Long-term Enteral Tube Feeding Decisions, The Bioethics Center, University of Alberta. Guidelines for health care professionals participating in decisions on long-term enteral tube feedings. Edmonton, Alberta: 1993.
8. Levinsky NG. Fluids and electrolytes. In Harrison's principles of internal medicine, 12th edn (ed. Wilson JD, Braunwald E, Isselbacher KJ, et al.). McGraw-Hill Inc. New York. 1991; 279–89.
9. Bruera E, MacDonald N. A study of a cardiovascular autonomic insufficiency in advanced cancer patients. Cancer Treatment Reports 1986: 70(12): 1383–7. Clin Invest Med 1985; 8(3); A168.
10. Breitbart W, Passik S. Psychiatric aspects of palliative care. In: The Oxford textbook of palliative medicine (ed. Doyle D, Hanks GW, MacDonald N). London: Oxford University Press, 1993: pp. 607–26.
11. Wright RR, Tono M, Pollycove M. Blood volume. Seminars Nucl Med 1975; 5(1): 63–78.
12. Natkunam A, Shek CC, Swaminathan R. Hyponatremia in a hospital population. J Med 1991; 22(2): 83–96.
13. Tang WW, Kaptein EM, Feinstein EI, Massry SG, Eben IF. Hyponatremia in hospitalized patients with the acquired immunodeficiency syndrome (AIDS and the AIDS-related complex). Americasn Journal of Medicine 1993: 94(2): 169–74.
14. Gross AJ, Steinberg SM, Reilly JG et al. A natriuretic factor and arginine vasopressin production in tumor cell lines from patients with lung cancer and their relationship to serum sodium. Cancer Res 1993; 53: 67–74.
15. Bliss JRDP, Battey JF, Linnoila RI et al. Expression of the atrial natriuretic factor gene in small cell lung cancer tumors and tumor cell lines. J Nat Cancer Inst 1990; 82(4): 305–10.
16. Rousseau P. Hyponatremia among older individuals. Southern Med J 1991; 84(9): 114–18.
17. Silver AJ. Aging and risks for dehydration. Cleveland Clin J Med 1990; 57(4): 341–4.
18. Southgate HJ, Burke BJ, Walters G. Body space measurements in the hyponatremia of carcinoma of the bronchus: evidence for the chronic 'sick cell' syndrome? Ann Clin Biochem 1992; 29: 90–5.
19. Wall BM, Crofton JT, Share L, Cooke CR. Chronic hyponatremia due to resetting of the osmostat in a patient with gastric carcinoma. 1992; 93: 223–8.
20. Flear CTG, Singh CM. Hyponatremia and sick cells. Br J Anesth 1973; 45: 976–94.
21. McConkey B. The effects of wasting on the body water. Clin Sci 1959; 18: 95–102.

22. McCance RA. Experimental sodium chloride deficiency in man. Proc R Soc Lond (Biol) 1936; 119: 245–68.
23. Gehi MM, Rosenthal RH, Fizette NB, Crowe LR, Webb WL. Psychiatric manifestations of hyponatremia. Psychosomatics 1981; 22(9): 739–43.
24. MacMillan HL, Gibson JC, Steiner M. Hyponatremia and depression. J Nerv Mental Dis 1990; 178(11): 720–1.
25. Zerwch JV. The dehydration question. Nursing 1983; 83: 47–51.
26. Micotech KC, Steinecker PH, Thomasma DC. Are intravenous fluids morally required for a dying patient? Arch Int Med 1983; 143: 975–8.
27. Siegler N, Weisbard HA. Against the emerging stream. Arch Int Med 1985; 145: 129–31.
28. Ahronhein JC, Gasner MR. The sloganism of starvation. Lancet 1990; 335: 278–9.
29. Billings JA. Comfort measures for the terminally ill. Is dehydration painful? J Am Geriat Soc 1985; 33: 808–10.
30. Millar RJ, Albright PG. What is the role of nutritional support and hydration in terminal cancer patients? Am J Hospice Care 1989; 5(6): 34–8.
31. Enck RE. Dehydration in the terminally ill (letter). Am J Hospice Care 1989; 5(5): 48.
32. Andrews MR, Levine AN. Dehydration in the terminal patient: perception of hospice nurses. Am J Hospice Care 1989; 6: 31–4.
33. Musgrave CF. Terminal dehydration. To give or not to give intravenous fluids? Cancer Nursing 1990; 13: 62–6.
34. Hamdy RC, Braverman AN. Ethical conflicts in long term care of the aged (letter). BMJ 180; 280(6215): 717.
35. Burge FI, King DB, Willison D. Intravenous fluids and the hospitalized dying: a medical last rite? Can Family Physician 1990; 86: 883–6.
36. Twycross RG. Symptom control: the problem areas. Palliat Mcd 1993; 7:1–8.
37. Andrews M, Bell ER, Smith SA et al. Dehydration in terminally ill patients. Is it appropriate palliative care? Postgrad Med 1993; 93: 201–8.
38. Yan E, Bruera E. Parenteral hydration of terminally ill cancer patients. J Palliat Care 1991; 7(3): 40–3.
39. Fraser J. Comforts of home: home care of the terminally ill. Can Family Physician 1990; 36: 977–81.
40. Burge Fl. Dehydration symptoms of palliative care cancer patients. J Pain Symptom Manage 1993; 8: 454–64.
41. MacKay A. Moehl T, Slotar S. The effect of body hydrations state on oral fluids. Diastema 1986; 14: 5–9.
42. Sullivan RJ. Accepting death without artificial nutrition or hydration. J Gen Int Med 1993; 8: 220–4.
43. Fainsinger R, Bruera E. Hypodermoclysis for symptom control vs the Edmonton Injector. J Palliat Care 1991: 7(4): 5–8.
44. Fainsinger R, MacEachern T, Miller MJ et al. The use of hypodermoclysis for rehydration in terminally ill cancer patients. J Pain Symptom Manage (in press).
45. Fainsinger RL, MacDonald SM. Letter to the Editor: accepting death without artificial nutrition or hydration. J Gen Int Med 1994; 9(2): 115–16.
46. Levinsky NG. Fluids and electrolytes. In: Harrison's principles of internal medicine, 12th edn (ed. Wilson JD, Braunwald E, Isselbacher KJ, et al.) New York: McGraw-Hill. 1991; 279–89.
47. Gopinathan PM, Pichan G, Sharma VM. Role of dehydration in heat stress induced variations in mental performance. Arch Environ Health 1988; 43: 15–17.
48. Shearer S. Dehydration and serum electrolyte changes in South African gold miners with heat disorders. Am J Indust Med 1990; 17: 225–39.
49. Burke AL, Daimond PL, Hulbert J et al. Terminal restlessness — its management and the role of midazolam. Med J Aust 1991; 155: 485–7.
50. Bruera E, Miller L, McCallion J, Macmillan, K, Krefting L, Hanson J. Cognitive failure

(CF) in patients with terminal cancer; a prospective study. J Pain Sympt Manag 1992; Vol 7(4): 192–5.

51. Grantham JJ. Acute renal failure. In: Cecil textbook of medicine 19th edn (ed. Wyngaarden JB, Smith LH, Bennett JC). Philadelphia: Saunders. 1992; 527–33.

52. Anderson RJ, Schrier RW. Acute renal failure. In Harrison's principles of internal medicine 12th edn (ed. Wilson JD, Braunwald E, Isselbacher KJ, et al.) New York: McGraw-Hill. 1991; 1144–50.

53. Neeser M, Ruedin P, REstellini JP. 'Thirst Strike': hypernatremia and acute renal failure in a prisoner who refused to drink. BMJ 1992; 304(6838): 1352.

54. Glare PA, Walsh TD, Pippenger CE. Normorphine, a neurotoxic metabolite? (Letter). Lancet 1990; 335 (8691): 725–6.

55. Pasternak FW, Bodnar RJ, Clark JA, Inturrisi CE. Morphine-6-glucuronide, a potent mu agonist. Life Sci 1987, 41(26): 2845–9.

56. Hagen NA, Foley KM, Cerbone DJ et al. Chronic nausea and morphine-6-glucuronide. J Pain Symptom Manage 1991; 6(3): 125–8.

57. Sear JW, Hand CW, Moore RA, McQuay HJ. Studies on morphine disposition: influence of renal failure on the kinetics of morphine and its metabolites. Br J Anaesth 1989; 62: 28–32.

58. Peterson GM, Randall CT, Paterson J. Plasma levels of morphine and morphine-glucuronides in the treatment of cancer pain: relationship to renal function and route of administration. Eur J Clin Pharmacol 1990; 38: 121–4.

59. Hanks GW, Hoskin PJ, Ahurne GW, Turner P. Explanation for potency of repeated oral doses of morphine? Lancet 1987; 2: 723–5.

60. De Conno F. Ventafridda V, Saiata L. Skin problems in advanced terminal cancer patients. J Pain Symptom Manage 1991; 6: 247–56.

61. MacDonald NJ, McConnell KN, Stephen MR et al. Hypernatremic dehydration in patients in a large hospital for the mentally handicapped. BMJ 1989; 229: 1426–29.

62. Sykes N. Constipation and diarrhea. In: (ed. Doyle D, Hanks G, MacDonald N). Oxford textbook of palliative medicine. New York: Oxford University Press. 1993; 299–310.

63. Back IN. Terminal restlessness in patients with advanced malignant disease. Palliat Med 1992; 6: 293–8.

64. Dunlop RJ. Is terminal restlessness sometimes drug induced? Palliat Med 1989; 3: 65–6.

65. Lichter I, Hunt E. The last 48 hours of life. J Palliat Care 1990; 6(4): 7–15.

66. Sullivan RJ. Accepting death without artificial nutrition or hydration (see coments). (Review). Response. J Gen Int Med 1994; 8(4): 220–4.

67. Green W. Setting boundaries for artificial feeding. Hastings Center Rep 1984; December: 14(6): 8–10.

68. Berger E. Nutrition by hypodermoclysis. J Am Geriat Soc 1984; 32: 199–203.

69. Bruera E, Legris MA, Kuehn N, Miller MJ. Hypodermoclysis for the administration of fluids and narcotic analgesics in patients with advanced cancer. J Pain Symptom Manage 1990; 5: 218–20.

70. Hays H. Hyopdermoclysis for symptom control in terminal cancer. Can Family Physician 1985; 31:1253–6.

71. Sethna RH. Hyopdermoclysis, an old idea resurrected. Modern Med Can 1986; 41: 8–12.

72. Doyle D. Care of the dying. In: Textbook of geriatric med and gerontology, 4th edn (ed. JC Brocklehurt, RC Tallis, RM Fillit). Edinburgh: Churchill Livingston, 1992; 1057–1061.

73. Molloy DW, Cunje A. Hypodermoclysis in the care of old adults. An old solution for new problems? Can Family Physician 1992; 38: 2038–43.

74. Collaud T, Rapin C. Dehydration and dying patients; study with physicians in French speaking Switzerland. J Pain Symptom Manage 1991; 6: 230–40.

75. Schen RJ, Singer-Edelstein M. Subcutaneous infusions in the elderly. J Am Gerial Soc 1981; 24: 583–5.

76. Schen RJ, Singer-Edelstein M. Hypodermoclysis (letter). JAMA 1983; 250: 1694–5.

77. Bruera E. Ambulatory infusion devices in the continuing care of patients with advanced diseases. J Pain Symptom Manage 1990; 5(5): 287–96.
78. Fainsinger RL, Miller M, Bruera E. Hypodermoclysis and dehydration. Can Family Physician 1992; 38: 2803.
79. Molloy DW. Response. Can Family Physician 1992; 38: 2805.
80. Gluck S. Hypodermoclysis revisited (letter). JAMA 1982; 248: 1310–11.
81. Gluck SM. Advantages of hypodermoclysis. J Am Gerial Soc 1984; 32: 691–2.
82. Constans T, Dutertre J, Froge E. Hypodermoclysis in dehydrated elderly patients: local effects with and without hyaluronidasc. J Palliat CAre 1991; 7(2): 10–12.
83. Toscani F. Is pallation medicine?' Ethical and epistemological problems. J Palliat Care 1991; 7(3): 33–9.

Note: The second part of this chapter is adapted, with permission, from Fainsinger R, Bruera E. The management of dehydration in terminally ill patients. J Palliat Care 1994; 10(3): 55–9.

8

Enteral and parenteral nutrition in cancer patients

Antonio Vigano and Eduardo Bruera

INTRODUCTION

Malnutrition and weight loss are frequent complication of malignant disease. (1, 2) As previously mentioned, malnutrition is associated with several complications in cancer patients such as lower performance status, decreased response rate to antineoplastic treatments, increased mortality, and symptom distress (including asthenia, anorexia, and chronic nausea). (3, 4)

Because of these factors, aggressive nutrition has been used widely in these patients.

The purpose of this chapter is to describe enteral and parenteral nutrition, the results of aggressive nutritional studies in cancer patients, some general guidelines for the use of those techniques, and areas of future research.

MALNUTRITION AND ARTIFICIAL NUTRITION IN CANCER PATIENTS

Previous reviews have extensively reported data on epidemiology and clinical consequences of malnutrition in cancer patient, which have been reported in Table 8.1. (5)

Table 8.1 Complications of cancer cachexia (4)

Reduced response to antineoplastic drug (1)
Diminished tolerance to radiation and chemotherapy (1)
Higher incidence of perioperative complications (6)
Decreased survival (4)
Higher incidence of symptoms related to cachexia (5)
Decreased performance status (3)

With the purpose of reversing those complications, several authors have tried to identify and treat cancer cachexia.

As discussed in Chapter 6, malnutrition in cancer patients may be perceived through the dietary history, (7, 8) quantization of a recent weight loss (within 3 months), physical examination, evaluation of specific laboratory tests, and knowledge of the anticipated method of treatment. (9) A 10% loss in current weight as compared to the usual patient's weight has been consistently associated with an increased risk of surgical complications (10) and a more limited survival. (11)

Clinical history with emphasis on weight loss, dietary patterns, and gastrointestinal (GI) symptomatology, in combination with thorough physical examination have been found in most cases as effective as objective measurements in identifying malnourished patients. (12)

Anthropometric and biochemical methods have been shown unreliable indicators of nutritional status in cancer patients due to the frequent changes related to the underlying malignancy, its treatments, and complications. (13) However, a serum transferrin level less than 150 mg/dl, and a serum albumin less than 3.4 g/dl are still considered reliable indicators of cancer malnutrition. (14)

Some antineoplastic treatments have been associated with a high risk of nutritional deterioration: radical resections within the oral cavity, the head–neck area, and the GI tract. Radiation therapy to the oval cavity or the pharynx and intense adjuvant therapy regimens with bone marrow transplantation are typical precursors of cancer cachexia. (9)

In summary, useful and widely accepted rules of thumb to select cancer patients suitable for artificial nutrition include an unintentional or unexplained loss of 10% or more of body weight, a serum albumin level less than 3.4 g/dl, a serum transferrin level less than 150 mg/dl, and an inadequate spontaneous oral intake (< 60% predicted nutrient requirements for more than one week). Any two of those criteria and the provision of intensive antineoplastic therapy may be an indication for nutritional support or therapy. (9, 15)

NUTRITIONAL APPROACH

Current nutritional therapies for malnutrition include specialized nutrition support such as enteral nutrition (EN) and total parental nutrition (TPN). While TPN remains the 'gold standard' for nutrition support, (16) EN is the first choice alternative to the oral route in patients with a functional gut. (17)

Enteral nutrition is generally considered less expensive, more practical, and associated with fewer major complications than TPN. More recently, unique advantages have been found for EN in maintaining GI structure and function. Without enterocyte absorption of nutrients, there is a lack of stimuli for mucosal cell growth and elaboration of trophic hormones. Intestinal atrophy consequently occurs with loss of organism homeostasis and altered integrity of the GI tract as a mechanical barrier to bacterial transmigration. (16) Although the clinical relevance of bacterial translocation is not completely known yet in humans, (18) the maintenance of GI mucosal integrity, permits a more rapid return to normal eating.

As a consequence of increasing use of EN, TPN has become more and more restricted to patients with a dysfunctional gut or to patients who refuse enteral tubes or in whom enteral tubes may be non-insertable and/or too harmful. A few elective indications for TPN in cancer patients will be reviewed in the following paragraphs.

ENTERAL NUTRITION

Delivery

Enteral feeding has been defined by the American Society of Parenteral and Enteral Nutrition as the provision of liquid formula diets into the GI tract orally or by means of feeding tubes. (17)

Patients who require enteral support have a functional gut but are unable to take adequate nutrients orally to prevent protein-caloric malnutrition.

Multiple, easy to perform techniques for delivery of nutrients into the stomach, duodenum, or jejunum are available. Routes of administration include nasogastric, esophagogastric, or pharyngogastric, nasoduodenal or nasojujenal, gastric, gastroenteric, or jejunal. (19) In the latter three sites, tubes may be placed through an open surgical procedure, endoscopically, or under laparoscopic or ultrasound guidance. (18) Gastrostomy and jujenostomy are usually performed through the endoscopic approach; they are particularly indicated in patients who are unable to eat or swallow such as in head and neck cancer. Patients with completely obstructing pharyngeal or oesophageal tumors may not be good candidates for endoscopic procedures because of the impossibility to pass the endoscope. In this case laparoscopic or ultrasound guided procedures may be good alternatives, in the absence of other contraindications to 'ostomies' (for example, ascities or previous abdominal surgery sequela). (20)

The Percutaneous endoscopic gastrostomy (PEG) and operative jejunostomy became the most popular techniques for enteral feeding. PEG is indicated for patients who require long-term feeding since it avoids the irritation of nasal tubes and the need of open abdominal surgery. In the occurrence of the latter procedure, a prophylactic jejunostomy tube may be placed in patient at high risk of nutritional deterioration, even without initiation of the nutritional support. (19) If tube feeding is likely to be needed for several months, traditional surgical gastrostomy is preferred as it is more comfortable and makes long-term nursing care easier. (21)

Gastric and jejunal feedings offer different advantages. In general, the latter is provided by a lower risk of aspiration. Due to the protection offered by the pyloric sphincter and the ligament of Treitz, the highest rate of aspiration is associated with delivery into the stomach and the lowest with delivery into the jejunum. (18)

The advantages of feeding into the stomach include ease of tube placement, physiologic similarity to normal GI function, the possibility of using hyperosmolar formula, and the option of continuous or bolus feeding which reduce patient care time. (20)

An important aspect of enteral nutrition is represented by the availability of new type of feeding tubes. Small-bore (8 to 10 French) and flexible nasoenteral tubes, have ameliorated patient tolerance. Made from biocompatible materials such as silicone or polyurethane, PEG or jejunostomy tubes are now more durable than Foley or Malecot catheters and eliminate the need for frequent replacement because of hardening or cracking. (22)

Nasogastric tubes are usually 91 cm long, while the 109 cm long tube with a tungsten weight is used for spontaneous or direct passage of the tip through the pylorus into the distal duodenum or upper jejunum. The placement is facilitated by an inner stylet that stiffens the catheter and documented by fluoroscopy or X-rays, prior to starting feeding.

The diameter of the tube is determined by the viscosity and osmolality of the formula. As a general rule, the smallest bore tube that allows the formula to flow without clogging should be used for greater patient acceptance. (15)

The composition and general nutrient profile of enteral formulas have become very sophisticated. Their description is beyond the scope of this chapter and many compendia are available to help in selection. (23, 24)

From a practical point of view, currently available enteral formulations may be divided in four categories: blenderized tube-feeding formulas, nutritionally complete commercial formulas, chemically defined formulas, and modular formulas. (25)

Blenderized tube feedings may be prepared with any food that can be blenderized such as meat, whole or skim milk, vegetables, fruit, and cereal. These formulas may be home-made or commercial preparations.

Caloric density and protein contents of those preparations may be easily increased by the addition of vegetable oils, corn syrup, modular formula, dry milk, or egg. There is, however, less flexibility in vitamin, mineral, and electrolyte content. Caloric concentrations of those formula vary from 0.6 to 1.3 kcal/ml. (15)

Blenderized food is usually less costly than commercial formulas, but presents several disadvantages. It has to be administered only by a large bore feeding tube, it may facilitate bacterial growth, it may not be homogenous, and it may be inconsistent in term of nutrient composition.

Nutritionally complete commercial formulas provide sterile, homogenous solutions that are easy to prepare, relatively inexpensive, and administered by small-bore feeding tubes. They contain approximately 1–1.5 kcal/ml and guarantee a fixed nutrient profile. Most are lactose free and flavored for oral supplementation.

Chemically defined formulas are commonly called elemental diets. The nutrients are provided in a pre-digested and readily absorbed form. Due to the presence of amino acids, those formulas are not palatable and deserved for tube feeding. They are useful for patients with digestive disturbances, such as post-radiation enteritis or pancreatic insufficiency. They are very low in residue, lactose free, and provide approximately 1 kcal/ml. Their main disadvantages are the cost and the high osmolality, which may cause fluid retention and secondary diarrhea. (26)

Modular formulas are prepared for patients with specific nutrient needs or organ dysfunction. They consist of core modules of protein, carbohydrate, fat, vitamin, and mineral mixture that are not nutritionally complete individually but can be used to modify other enteral formulas and tailor them for specific needs. (15)

The initial patient's medical assessment, will aid in the selection of enteral formulas. Either physicians or nutrition therapists should investigate the presence of electrolytes imbalances, diabetes, congestive heart failure, pancreatic insufficiency, liver disease, and lung disease and the presence of specific needs due to the neoplastic disease and/or its treatment. (27) Pre-digested formulas, such as elemental or modular diets, are indicated in cancer patients with maldigestion (for example, pancreatic insufficiency, biliary or pancreatic diversion, etc.) or malabsorption (for example, short-bowel syndrome). Patients with liver disease, may benefit from formulas enriched in branched-chain amino acids, while in the presence of renal failure, a low protein content may be advisable. A low carbohydrate formula may facilitate control glucose in diabetic or insulin-resistant patients; congestive heart failure, ascites, oliguric renal insufficiency, or pulmonary edema are the main indications for fluid restricted formulas.

In severely malnourished cancer patients, formulas enriched with branched chain amino acids, arginine, omega–3 fatty acids, and glutamine, may have a role in reducing patient morbidity, (28) as it will be discussed later in this chapter.

For food feeding, most protocols suggest the following steps: (29, 30)

1. Prior to formula administration, verify all tube placements by X-ray and flush with 25 ml water to confirm patency.

2. Begin with continuous administration by volumetric pump at 10 ml/h.

3. Elevate the head of the bed 30 degrees or more, while administering the enteral diet.

4. Use full-strength diets.

5. Increase gradually 10ml/h every 24 hours in the most critically ill and faster (for example, 8 or 12 hours) in the less severely ill patients. Usually final rates are, for continuous feeding 50–60 cc/h, for discontinuous administration (night cycles, 8–12 hours) 100–120 ml/h and for bolus feeding (syringe or gravity drip) 250ml per bolus.

6. Monitor tolerance when formula administration begins (see following paragraph for complications).

7. Check gastric residuals at least every 4 hours only if intragastric feeding is used. If the total volume of the residual exceeds 50% of the delivered formula or 150 ml, discontinue the infusion for 2 hours, or reduce the rate of the formula by half. After 2 hours recheck for residual: if the volume is still exceeding normal ranges, use metoclopramide (10 mg IV or enteral four times a day) or cisapride (10 mg orally four times a day), to increase gastric motility. The residual check is not indicated in post-pylorically fed patients.

8. Reassess for tube-feeding tolerance on a daily basis.

Contra-indications and complications

Enteral nutrition is contra-indicated in any condition which results in intestinal dismotility or mechanical obstruction. It is also contra-indicated in any condition in which the feeding itself may have a negative impact on the recovery process such as upper intestinal bleeding, intestinal fistula, and acute pancreatitis. Finally, enteral feeding is not appropriate in situations such as a severe malabsorption state or in the presence of vomiting and diarrhea in which the feeding may aggravate fluid depletion or other complication. (18)

Complications of enteral feeding include GI disturbances, metabolic abnormalities, and mechanical difficulties as outlined in Table 8.2. (20)

Table 8.2 Common complications associated with enteral feeding

GASTROINTESTINAL
  Nausea and vomiting
Aspiration
Diarrhea
Constipation

METABOLIC	MECHANICAL
Dehydration	Occluded or clogged feeding tube
Elevated/depressed serum electrolytes	Nasal irritation or erosion
Hyperglycemia	Tube displacement

Diarrhea, aspiration, and occlusion of the feeding tube are frequent complications of EN in cancer patients.

Diarrhea may be defined as > 500 ml stool output over a 24 hour period or more than three stools per day. (31) It is usually secondary to a high osmotic load (> 1000 mOs/kg), which may occur from either nutrients or medication which are added to the tube-feeding formula. Medications usually may not only increase formula osmolality but also irritate the GI tract and stimulate its motility: sorbitol containing elixir, magnesium antacids, cimetidine, potassium and phosphorus supplements, quinidine compounds, lactulose, and various laxatives may be suspected of either causing or contributing consistently to the diarrheic syndrome.

Diarrhea may be common in enterally fed cancer patients who receive antibiotics, primarily due to altered colonization of the GI tract, or are affected by enteritis, as a result of post-chemotherapy or radiotherapy enteritis.

Test stool cultures for ova and parasites with a Clostridium difficile toxin assay, may useful in identifying the offending pathogens.

The proper treatment of diarrhea will depend on the cause; if the diarrhea is caused by the formula, since no single formula is associated with a lower incidence of diarrhea, it is advisable to change to a formula with a lower osmolality (no greater than 500 mOsm) or to a fibre-containing formula. If the diarrhea persists after those procedures, a switch to an elemental or peptide-based formula is suggested. (27) The management of an idiopathic diarrhea usually relies on a judicious use of hypomobility agent such as Lomotil, deodorized tincture of opium, or psyllium. Failure of the latter treatments may represent a definite indication for TPN. (31)

Aspiration feeding is a complication observed only in the intragastrically fed patient and is generally due to delayed gastric emptying. Major causes of the latter phenomenon in cancer patients are autonomic failure, lytes imbalance (for example, hypercalcemia and hypokalemia) diabetic gastroparesis, surgical repairs, cancer progression (for example, liver enlargement secondary to metastatization, intestinal obstruction, visceral carcinosis, etc.), and drugs with anticholinergic properties (tricyclics, narcotics, anti-acids, etc.). The formula is unlikely to be a contributing factor unless any of the following characteristics are present: osmolality (> 650 mOs/kg), fat (long-chain triglycerides), content (> 10% total calories), or rate (patient receiving more than 25–30 Kcal/kg).

Methods for detecting and treating high gastric residuals secondary to delayed emptying have been previously mentioned; if the problem persists after those procedures, a post-pyloric type of feeding (for example, a percutaneous gastrostomy–jejunostomy or a surgical jejunostomy) may be indicated. (31)

Whenever a complication is suspected to be secondary to increased gastric residuals (for example, aspiration pneumonia), the addition of few drops of methylene blue to the feeding formula will be helpful in tracing the route of the formula.

The last but certainly not the least occurring complication with enteral feeding of cancer patients, is the tube clogging. Better management of this complication is its prevention, by always flushing the tube with 20 ml warm water when feeding is stopped, or interrupted, before and after medicines.

In providing drugs via the feeding tube, we would also recommend the following steps. (32)

1. Only electrolytes, vitamins and minerals should be added directly to the tube-feeding formula (for example, NaCI, KCI, $NaOH_3$, $CaCI_2$, multivitamin, etc.).

2. Bolus administer other medications (finely crushed and mixed with 20 ml warm water).

3. Avoid administering medications (non-electrolytes) via a jejunostomy, because they are usually absorbed in the duodenum.

4. Do not give enteric-coated or sustained-release medications via any feeding tube.

5. Avoid syrups high in alcohol, which may cause coagulation of the enteral formula.

If true clogging occurs, it may be caused generally by proteins (the major component of enteral diets which likely tends to coagulate) and/or medications. Papain 2.5% (an enzyme derived from pineapple) and/or Coca-cola may be instilled in the feeding tube, allowing a 30-minute permanence of the solution (1–5 ml) and flushing the tube afterwards, with warm water. If the 'chemical approach' fails (two or three attempts are usually advised) a guidewire (0.35 mm) may by gently inserted to clear the obstruction.

Finally, careful attention to the patient metabolic status and fluid and electrolyte balance is necessary to avoid metabolic complications, which however seem not as common in the cancer population as they are among the acutely ill. (20)

Patients who receive enteral feeding require the same careful monitoring as those who receive parenteral nutrition. Monitoring is best accomplished by employing protocols, standard orders, and follow-up of patients by a nutrition support service.

TOTAL PARENTERAL NUTRITION

Delivery

Total parenteral nutrition (TPN) can be defined as the provision of all nutrients necessary to sustain life intravenously, without using the intestinal tract. (19) TPN has been also termed as parenteral nutrition, hyperalimentation, intravenous nutrition, intravenous feeding, and intravenous alimentation.

TPN is recognized as the primary route of nutrient delivery for patients with intestinal failure (for example, after massive small bowel resection) or in whom EN is contra-indicated (for example, ileus or bowel obstruction, fistulae, nausea, and vomiting); TPN is also indicated when rapid nutrition repletion is necessary. (33)

Intravenous nutrition may deliver all known essential nutrients in their optimal amounts (complete or total parenteral nutrition) or it may be partial or incomplete, with deficits in calories, protein or electrolytes, and minerals. Although special formulas have been developed for the patient with renal, hepatic, and pulmonary failure, no specific formula is used for the cancer patient. (15)

The hypertonic nutrient solution most commonly used for TPN in cancer patients parallels a normal diet and consists of 15–25% dextrose, 4–5% crystalline amino acids, 10% fat emulsion, electrolytes, and vitamins. Each unit of base solution provides approximately 5.25–6 g nitrogen and 900–1000 calories in 1000–1100 ml of water. (15)

The description of specific nutrient requirements is beyond our scope. From a practical point of view, fluid requirements for normal maintenance can be estimated from either body weight (30 ml/kg) or body surface area (1400 ml/m^2) and adjusted for existing deficits and ongoing excessive losses. Caloric requirements are calculated at around 35 kcal/kg/day for maintenance and 45 kcal/kg/day for anabolism. The daily provision of 10 g of nitrogen or 62.5 g of protein (1 g of nitrogen = 6.25 g of protein) prevents protein malnutrition in most adults. (15) In cancer patients, nitrogen requirements per day should be provided in a ratio of 1 g of nitrogen to 125–150 calories.

Among electrolytes, the daily requirements are as follows: sodium 60–120 mEq, potassium 60–100 mEq, chloride 60–120 mEq, magnesium 8–10 mEq, calcium 200–400 mg, and phosphorus 300–400 mg. (15)

Delivery of TPN may be via a central or peripheral vein. Peripheral venous access is usually performed through the basilic vein in the antecubital fossa. The peripheral route for parenteral nutrition is easier and less invasive than the central one. However, the administration of hypertonic solutions into low blood flow vessels causes severe burning and the rapid development of thrombophlebitis. (34) The standard solutions administered through the peripheral veins are usually less concentrated but also less caloric (~0.5 kcal/ml) than the solutions infused through central veins. They need to be delivered in big volumes and, in the case of TPN, supplemented by the infusion of 20% fat emulsions. (35) The peripheral parenteral nutrition is therefore used only for short periods of time (< 10 days), for non-fluid-restricted patients and in pediatric patients. (25)

The most common vascular access used for TPN is a percutaneously placed subclavian vein catheter. This technique may provide easy placement and dressing management, allows the patient's arm and neck free of normal motion, and has a lower rate of complications. (36)

The second most used route of venous catheterization for TPN is the internal jugular vein: among the cancer population, this access may be preferred to the subclavian vein in emphysematous patients, where there is an increased risk of a tension pneumothorax, in the patient with a coagulopathy or thrombocytopenia, where a vascular damage may be more easily controlled with direct pressure in the neck, and in patients whose venous anatomy or thrombotic occlusion makes it difficult to incannulate the superior vena cava from the subclavian access. (37)

The central venous access allows the administration of hypertonic solutions and the long-term placement of catheters. Among those, the polyurethane catheters are currently preferred because of their lower thrombogenicity. Double- or triple-lumen catheters are also available, with one port for TPN and other ports for blood drawing, antibiotic administration, or chemotherapy administration. (38) Although a 15-year survival of a Broviac catheter used for home TPN has been described in an elderly patient affected by Crohn's disease, (39) multiple lumen catheters are not routinely implemented due to a greater incidence of catheter-related infections associated with their use. (40)

Complications and contra-indications of TPN

Complications of TPN may be mechanical, metabolic, infectious, and not obviously related to TPN, as reported in Table 8.3. Mechanical and septic complications are related to obtaining and maintaining a route of vascular access. The description of the technical procedures to avoid those complications is beyond our purposes; however the following guidelines have been suggested to reduce catheter-related sepsis in a patient who might have been transferred/admitted to a medical or surgical ward for receiving TPN: (41)

Table 8.3 Common complications of TPN

MECHANICAL	SEPTIC
Pneumothorax	Contamination of the catheter
Malpositioning of the catheter	Sepsis
Thrombosis of the central vein	
METABOLIC	NOT OBVIOUSLY RELATED TO TPN
Volume overload	Increase of all infectious complications
Hyper/hypoglycemia	Higher mortality rate in cancer patients
Electolyte imbalance	
Essential micronutrient deficiencies	
Hepatic steatosis	
Cholestasis	
Pre-renal azotemia	
Excessive CO^2 production	
Metabolic bone disease	

1. Set a protocol for regular TPN monitoring.

2. 'Watchdog' TPN nurse.

3. Aseptic technique in insertion and in routine management.

4. Catheter use for nutrients only.

5. Avoid multilumen catheter.

6. Sterile solutions with laminar flow technique in preparation.

7. Tubing and dressing changes every 48 hours.

8. Avoid prophylactic antibiotics or antibiotic flushes.

9. Avoid routine changes of catheters without a specific indication.

10. Removal of catheters for infection at skin sites (positive skin cultures with a microorganisms concentration greater than $1000/cm^3$).

11. Use soft, non-thrombogenic catheters, preferably silicone elastomer or polyurethane.

12. Privilege insertion techniques with minimal trauma.

13. Add heparin (1–3 U/ml) to TPN solution.

Metabolic complications are caused by inadequate solution formulation and monitoring, frequently aggravated by some underlying metabolic abnormalities intrinsic to the patient and/or to his disease processes. (36)

The incidence of those complications is often dependent on the skills of the health care givers. The implementation of the nutritional support team, composed of a physician, dietician, nurse, and pharmacist, and the use of appropriate and standardized protocols for the administration of TPN and patient monitoring, significantly reduced complications, enhanced quality of nutritional care, and cost savings. (42)

An increase of infectious complications such as wound infections, abdominal infections, and pneumonias not related to intravenous line sepsis have been reported in patients receiving TPN. (43, 44) In cancer trials, TPN has been also associated with a higher mortality rate. (45) In the pathogenesis of those phenomena, which is still unclear, the increased permeability to bacteria and toxins secondary to the gut mucosal atrophy, which has been demonstrated in animals receiving TPN, the overgrowth of certain enteric bacilli due to simple intestinal obstruction and the general impairment of the immune system with a specific deficit of intestinal secretory IgA may play an important role by enhancing bacterial translocation. (46)

TPN is contra-indicated whenever there is an immediate problem that precludes its safe and effective administration (for example, coagulopathy, marked pulmonary emphysema, previous neck thoracic radiotherapy, operations, or central venous catheter placement) and the gut is functioning and available for EN. (36)

Other contra-indications for TPN are relative and include its use to prolong life in a terminally ill patient. (47)

EFFECTS OF NUTRITIONAL SUPPLEMENTATION IN CANCER PATIENTS

Although the clinical and prognostic implications of cancer cachexia are clear, the outcomes of aggressive and technologically sophisticated nutrition are still controversial (Table 8.4).

Table 8.4 Possible effects of nutritional support in cancer patients

---

Improved survival (limited evidence) (3, 44)
Improved tumor response after chemotherapy (limited evidence) (45, 49, 50)
Decreased toxicity from chemotherapy (minimal evidence) (45)
Decreased surgical complications (few data) (51, 54)
Decreased toxicity from radiotherapy (insufficient data) (15)
Increased tumor growth (indirect observations) (56)
Better quality of life (supporting data lacking) (57)

The nutritional support in cancer patients may accrue weight and improve lean body mass and nearly all components of metabolism, but seldom reverses completely cachexia. (3) Furthermore, since most cancer patients die from causes other than cachexia alone, nutritional support may have a limited impact on their prognosis.

In terms of prolonged survival or reduced toxicity from cancer chemotherapy, minimal or no apparent benefit has consistently been shown in the group that received TPN as compared with either nourished or malnourished control patients receiving standard oral nutrition. (45)

A position paper from the American College of Physicians was published following those data, which concluded that parenteral nutrition support is associated with net harm, and no condition can be defined in which such treatment appear to be of benefit'. (48)

An important exception to those observations may be represented by the finding of improved disease-free interval and overall survival with the use of TPN in patients undergoing bone-marrow transplantation. (49)

In a further prospective randomized trial of patients receiving a bone-marrow transplant, TPN was not found superior to enteral feeding and was recommended only in patients who demonstrated intolerance to enteral feeding. (50)

Controversial data support the use of perioperative nutritional support as a routine practice in unselected cancer patients undergoing major surgery. (51, 52) While trials with post-operative TPN have not shown consistent reductions in complications or mortality, studies dealing with pre-operative TPN administered for GI surgery, showed a reduction in crude morbidity ranging from 7 to 21% among artificially nourished cancer patients. (52, 53) The latter figure was shown by Fan *et al.* (52) in 124 patients undergoing resection of hepatocellular carcinoma: besides a consistent morbidity reduction, due to fewer septic complications, those authors also showed a reduction in the requirements for diuretic agents to control ascites, less weight loss after hepatectomy, and less deterioration of liver function in the patients who underwent perioperative nutritional support and were affected by underlying cirrhosis. In another study by the Veterans Affairs Total Parenteral Nutritional Cooperative Study Group, (54) 395 malnourished patients (> 65% with cancer) who required laparatomy or non-cardiac thoracotomy, were randomly assigned to receive either perioperative TPN or no nutritional support. While the rates of major complications and of mortality were similar in the two groups, in the sub group of the severely malnourished (5% of the sample), patients who received TPN had a 38% of reduction in non-infectious complications (for example, anastomotic leak or bronchopleural fistulae), without a concomitant increase in infectious complications.

The study confirmed the lack of benefit of TPN in borderline malnourished patients, provided strong evidence against its clinical efficacy in mildly or moderately malnourished patients, and suggested a potential benefit of TPN in severely malnourished patients.

A study based on cost–benefit analysis (monetary cost of a beneficial therapy related to the value of the benefits produced), cost-effectiveness analysis (benefit achieved related to the monetary cost to achieve it), and the effect size estimation (quantization of the magnitude of benefit for an effective therapy), has led to an interesting sensitivity analysis for pre-operative nutritional support among GI cancer patients. (37) Presuming that the occurrence of major complications, such as sepsis, anastomotic leak, renal failure, or intra-abdominal abscess, may cost more than $55 000 and accounting for a morbidity reduction of 13%, a 10-day hospitalization for pre-operative TPN is cost-saving ($2500 per patient) if the TPN is given incidentally or cost-neutral if the patient is hospitalized only for the administration of TPN. On the other hand, if the value taken in account for morbidity reduction is 7%, this reduction in complications may cost approximately $2000 if TPN is given incidentally and $5000 if it is not. Although not clinically tested, EN always seems to provide a consistent saving.

Further trials are needed in sub groups of high-risk patients such as severely malnourished cancer patients having major surgery or patients with complications which result in prolonged period of inadequate nutritional intake. It may also be interesting to assess the possible role of the tube feeding, rather than testing only the the TPN. (55)

An insufficient number of cases have been evaluated to establish the efficacy of nutritional support in patients receiving radiation therapy. (15)

Some evidence in animal studies and indirect observations in cancer patients suggest that TPN may increase tumor growth. At the present time, this possibility does not appear to be a clear contra-indication to using TPN in patients affected by malignant disease. (56)

Finally, the impact of supplement nutrition has not yet been considered on meaningful variables for the cancer patient such as symptom control (pain, nausea etc), psychologic, and social functioning. (57)

CLINICAL GUIDELINES FOR NUTRITIONAL SUPPORT IN CANCER PATIENTS

In clinical practice and in the cost-effectiveness studies previously mentioned, it is possible to see areas of potential benefit from nutritional support. However, with those few exceptions previously mentioned (bone marrow transplantation and pre-operative TPN), there are no clear suggestions from the literature that nutritional support effectively improves complications of malnutrition in cancer patients.

EN and TPN have been shown to reverse malnutrition partially but not to combat cancer: (56) any lasting benefit of nutritional therapy has been always related to the effectiveness of antineoplastic treatment. With that premise, a recent consensus conference of the European Association for Palliative Care (47) has suggested a step-wise approach (Table 8.5) in the process of decision making for or against artificial feeding of cancer patients.

Table 8.5 Steps in the decision making of nutritional support of cancer patients

---

Step 1: to collect the key elements for a decision
   Point 1: define the oncological clinical condition
   Point 2: define the expected survival
   Point 3: hydration and nutritional status assessment
   Point 4: define symptoms
   Point 5: define nutrients intake
   Point 6: define the psychological attitude of the patients
   Point 7: define the gut function and the route of giving nutrients or water
   Point 8: define the availability of the health service to provide the therapy
Step 2: making the decision
Step 3: validate the indication

Following these steps, patients, relatives, and care givers with different social, cultural, scientific backgrounds can define individualized standards and goals for nutrition.

Cancer patients may benefit from nutritional support when they are malnourished and they are undergoing antineoplastic treatments with high nutritional morbidity. (53, 54)

Even in the absence of effective curative treatments, EN can be useful in some patients who are severely hypophagic because of cancer of the upper GI tract. They may be unable to swallow properly, but still have a normal appetite and a good performance status. (5)

In contrast, there may be patients in a terminal stage of their cancer with malignant bowel obstruction, who are confined to bed and require intensive pharmacologic therapy to control symptoms, such as pain, delirium, or dyspnea. In those patients a nutritional support is usually contra-indicated. (47)

In between these extreme cases, there are many intermediate situations where an indication for nutritional support may be more doubtful. In those situations, patients and family should be directly and actively involved in the decision-making process.

Whenever a decision regarding the feeding of cancer patients is taken, this needs to be re-evaluated periodically or with the onset of a new event that may change some of the key elements of the decision-making process. The therapeutic/palliative outcomes from nutritional support should be monitored in practice, according to the expected goals. In the palliative care setting for example, an unwanted prolongation of patient's survival should be balanced by an acceptable quality of their life. (47) The new placement of tracheostomy may complicate a TPN, while, with a sudden deterioration of a patient's conditions, nutritional support may become neither desirable nor attainable anymore. (36)

Parenteral nutrition has a complication rate of 15%, a high cost estimated at $10 000.00 per patient (44) and is not considered any different and/or superior to EN in reversing malnutrition. (50) Therefore, enteral feeding of cancer patients is favored when it is possible and not contra-indicated.

General suggestions regarding caloric and protein requirements have been given previously. Other macro- and micronutrients are calculated on an individual basis.

At present, rational outcomes of nutritional support in cancer patients may include amelioration of malnutrition, improvement of immunocompetence and body image. (3, 36) The correction or the prevention of the malnutrition symptoms such as asthenia, anorexia, psychosis/depression, cognitive impairment, loss of autonomy, etc., are still anecdotal. (57)

FUTURE RESEARCH

The nutritional management presented in the previous sections of this chapter, has been shown to provide the necessary nutrients to cancer patients. However, the latter are often unable to use those nutrients to reverse cancer-induced malnutrition. (56)

An improved knowledge of pathophysiology of cancer cachexia, which has been presented elsewhere in this book (Chapter 1), has resulted in defining critical components, which may not only exacerbate malnutrition but also limit nutritional support outcomes. Therefore, 'nutritional manipulation' represents the real challenge of the future: it consists practically in the modification of the tumor-bearing host metabolism by the administration of specific substrates and hormones, which are listed in Table 8.6. (58)

Table 8.6 Nutritional manipulation: proposed agents (58)

Agents	Proposed mechanism of action
Arginine, RNA, and omega–3 fatty acids (59–61)	Stimulate immune system, increase production of anabolic hormones
Glutamine (62)	Protect GI integrity
Hydrazine sulfate (63)	Decreases glyconeogenesis
Tumor necrosis factor (TNF) antibodies, and soluble TNF receptors (67, 68)	TNF binding and deactivation
Insulin, growth hormones, and anabolic steroids (70–73)	Decrease proteolysis and lipolysis, increase protein synthesis and appetite

Arginine, RNA, and omega–3 fatty acids may reverse immunocompetence impairment associated with cancer cachexia. (59) Arginine-enriched feedings have been found to stimulate the immune system, wound-healing, and the secretion of anabolic hormones such as growth hormone and insulin in tumor-bearing animals which often resulted in their increased survival. (60, 61)

RNA and omega–3 fatty acids have been shown to improve immunologic function in animal models by enhancing maturation of T cells and decreasing prostaglandin E2 production, respectively. (59)

Another amino acid, glutamine, has been found to be a major fuel for the GI mucosal cell in animals: in humans, the glutamine supplementation in TPN could reduce the stomatitis and enteritis associated with chemotherapy and the gut atrophy, mainly responsible for the previously mentioned bacterial translocation. (62)

Although very promising, manipulation solutions by those substrates are very expensive and their real advantage over conventional diets is still controversial in humans. (15, 55)

Hydrazine sulfate (HS) has a definitive role in limiting glyconeogenesis which is disproportionably enhanced in cancer cachexia. Besides a positive action on glucose intolerance and excessive glucose production in cancer patients, (63) HS did not show to ameliorate consistently the nutritional status in randomized, placebo-controlled studies. (64, 65)

Cytokines such as TNF and interleukin (IL) -1 and -6, are important mediators of cancer cachexia by accompanying progressive tumor growth, normal tissue destruction, and the host's inability to undergo cancer treatment and adequate nutritional support. (66)

However, clinical outcomes from the use of those substances in humans may be limited by the fact that cytokines are produced only by a minority of tumor types. (69)

Some experimental and human data have suggested that hormonal manipulation by insulin, growth hormone, and anabolic steroids may be beneficial in the treatment of cancer cachexia.

Insulin was found to improve cachectic parameters in animals with tumors or treated with tumor necrosis factor. (70) In those animals, insulin combined with antineoplastic therapy such as surgical resection or chemotherapy, also improved the tumor response rate to those therapies. (71) In humans the insulin levels have been considered as predictors of the ability of TPN to improve the body cell mass in cachectic patients. (72)

Administration of recombinant growth hormone or anabolic steroids in cancer patients, has been also shown to improve the host's ability to retain nitrogen and phosphorus during TPN and decrease proteolysis, respectively, both in animals and in humans. (73) However, further studies are needed to validate the clinical effectiveness of those hormones in reversing complications of neoplastic malnutrition. (56)

The other specific anti-anorexia treatments, such as anti-emetics, cyproheptadine, cannabinoids, and megestrol acetate have been previously reviewed (7) and will be mentioned elsewhere in this book (Chapter 9).

In summary, future trends in nutritional therapy are heading toward possible reversals or manipulations of metabolic mechanisms that lead to cancer cachexia, while providing adequate nutrients for the maintenance of the host nutritional status.

REFERENCES

1. DeWys WD, Begg C, Lavin PT *et al*. Prognostic effect of weight loss prior to chemotherapy in cancer patients. Am J Med 1980;69:491–97.
2. Warren S. The immediate cause of death in cancer patients. Am J Med 1932;184:610–13.
3. Bozzetti F. Effects of artificial nutrition on the nutritional status of cancer patients. J Parent Ent Nutri 1989; 13(4):406–20.
4. Bruera E, McDonald RN. Nutrition in patients with advanced cancer: an update and review of our experience. J Pain Symptom Manage 1988; 3:133–40.
5. Vigano A, Watanabe S, Bruera E. Anorexia and cachexia in advanced cancer patients. Cancer Surveys 1994; 21:99–115.
6. Smale B, Mullen J, Buzby G and Rosato E. The efficacy of nutritional assessment and support in cancer surgery. Cancer 1984; 47: 2375–81.

7. Bruera A, Chadwick S, Cowan L, *et al*. Caloric intake assessment in advanced cancer patients: a comparison of three methods. Cancer Treat Report, 1986; 70:981–3.
8. Corli O, Cozzolino A, Battaiotto Bernoni M, Gallina A. A new method of food intake quantification: application to the care of the patients. J Pain Symptom Manage 1992; 7(1):12–7.
9. Ollenschlager G, Konkol K, Modder B. Indications for and results of nutritional therapy in cancer patients. Recent Results in Cancer Research, 1988; nutritional therapy in cancer patients. Recent Results Cancer Res 1988;108:172–84.
10. Studley HO. Percentage of weight loss: a basic indicator of surgical risk in patients with chronic peptic ulcer. J Am Med Assoc 1936;106:458–60.
11. DeWys WD. Anorexia in cancer patients. Cancer Res 1977;37:2354–8.
12. Baker JP, Detsky AS, Wesson DE. Nutritional assessment: a comparison of clinical judgement and objective measurements. New Engl J Med 1982;306:969.
13. Sclafani LM, Brennan MF. Nutritional support in the cancer patient. In: Total parenteral nutrition, 2nd edn (ed. Fisher JE). Boston: Little Brown, 1991;323–46.
14. Hickey MS. Nutritional assessment guidelines. In: Handbook of enteral, parenteral and ARC/AIDS nutritional therapy (ed. Hickey MS). St Louis: Mosby–Year Book, 1992;1–23.
15. Daly JM, Torosian MH. Nutritional support. In: Cancer principle and practice of oncology, 4th edn (ed. DeVita VT, Hellman S, Rosenberg SA). Philadelphia: Lippincott, 1993;2480–501.
16. Shikora SA. Requirements for patients receiving enteral nutrition. In: Enteral nutrition (ed. Borlase BC, Bell SJ, Blackburn GL, Armour Forse R). New York: Chapman & Hall, 1994;37–46.
17. American Society for Parenteral and Enteral Nutrition (ASPEN), Board of Directors. Guidelines for the use of enteral nutrition in the adult patient. J Parent Ent Nutr 1987;11:435–9.
18. Saunders C, Nishikawa R, Wolfe B. Surgical nutrition: a review. J R Coll Surgeons Edin 1993;38:195–204.
19. Silberman H. Parenteral and enteral nutrition, 2nd edn. Norwalk: Appleton and Lange, 1989;130–44.
20. Guenter P, Susan J, Jacobs DO, Rombeau JL. Administration and delivery of enteral nutrition. In: Clinical nutrition: enteral nutrition, 2nd edn (ed. Rombeau JL, Caldwell MD). Philadelphia: Saunders 1993;512–36.
21. Deveney K. Endoscopic gastrostomy and jejunostomy. In: Clinical nutrition: enteral nutrition, 2nd edn (ed. Rombeau JL, Caldwell MD). Philadelphia: Saunders, 1993;512–36.
22. Ottery FD. More than an apple a day. A practical approach to nutritional supplement of the cancer patient. In: Current problems in cancer supportive care in oncology (ed. Ozols RF). St Louis: Mosby–Year Book Inc., 1992;367–78.
23. Shronts E, Havala T. Formulas. In: Nutrition support handbook (ed. Teasley-Strausburg K, Cerra F, Lehmann S, Shronts E). Cincinnati: Harvey Whitney Books Co, 1992;147–86.
24. McBurney M Russell C, Young LS. Formulas. In: Clinical nutrition: parenteral nutrition, 2nd edn (ed. Rombeau, JL, Caldwell, MD). Philadelphia: Saunders, 1993;512–36.
25. Daly JM, Thom AK. Neoplastic disease. In: Nutrition and metabolism in patient care. (ed. Kinney JM, Jeejeeboy KN, Graham LH, Owen OE). Philadelphia: Saunders, 1988;567–87.
26. Page CP, Hardin TC. Selection of liquid formula diet. In: Nutritional assessment and support: a primer. (ed. Page CP, Hardin TC). Baltimore: Williams & Wilkins, 1989;99–110.
27. Pasulka PS, Crockett C. Selecting enteral products. In: Enteral nutrition, (ed. Borlase BC, Bell SJ, Blackburn GL, Armour Forse R). New York: Chapman & Hall, 1994;115–41.
28. Daly JM, Lieberman MD, Goldine MS et al. Enteral nutrition with supplemental arginine, RNA and omega–3 fatty acids in patients after operation: immunologic, metabolic, and clinical outcome. Surgery 1992;112(1) 56–67.
29. Heanue P. Enteral feeding formulas and administrative techniques In: Enteral nutrition, (ed. Borlase BC, Bell SJ, Blackburn GL, Armour Forse R). New York: Chapman & Hall, 1994;173–80.

30. Hickey MS. Enteral nutritional therapy guidelines. In: Handbook of enteral and parenteral, and ARC/AIDS nutritional therapy (ed. Hickey MS). St Louis: Mosby-Year Book, 1992;34–100.

31. Shanti T. Gastrointestinal complications: diarrhea and high gastric residuals. In: Enteral nutrition (ed. Borlase BC, Sell SJ, Blackburn GL, Armour Forse R). New York: Chapman & Hall, 1994;188–92.

32. Thibault A. Care of feeding tubes. In: Enteral nutrition, (ed. Borlase BC, Bell SJ, Blackburn GL, Armour Forse R). New York: Chapman & Hall, 1994;197–8.

33. Payne-James JJ, Khawaja HT. First choice for total parenteral nutrition: the peripheral route. J Parent Ent Nutr 1993;17(5):468–78.

34. Grant JP. Catheter access. In: Clinical nutrition: parenteral nutrition, 2nd edn (ed. Rombeau JL, Caldwell MD). Philadelphia: Saunders, 1993;512–36.

35. Hickey MS. Parenteral nutritional therapy guidelines. In: Handbook of enteral and parenteral, and ARC/AIDS nutritional therapy (ed. Hickey MS). St Louise: Mosby-Year Book, 1992;110–83.

36. Page CP, Hardin TC. Complications of parenteral feeding. In: Nutritional assessment and support: a primer (ed. Page CP, Hardin TC). Baltimore: Williams & Wilkins, 1989;99–110.

37. Flowers JF, Ryan JA, Gough JA. Catheter-related complications of total parenteral nutrition In: Total parenteral nutrition, 2nd edn (ed. Fisher JE). Boston: Little Brown, 1991;25–46.

38. Pine RW, Crocker KS, Steffee WP. Triple lumen central venous catheter. Nutrition in clinical practice. 1986:1:90–6.

39. Buchman AL, Ament ME. Fifteen-year survival of a Broviac catheter used for home parenteral nutrition. J Parent Ent Nutr 1993;17(5):489.

40. Sherman RA, Flynn NM, Bradford M et al. Multilumen catheter sepsis and educational process to combat it. Am J Infect Control 1988;16:31a–4a.

41. Flowers JF, Ryan JA, Gough JA Catheter-related complications of total parenteral nutrition In: Total parenteral nutrition, 2nd edn (ed. Fisher JE). Boston: Little Brown, 1991;25–46.

42. Lipman TO. Efficacy and safety of total parenteral nutrition. Nutrition 1990;6(4):319–28.

43. Buzby GP. Results of the V.A. Cooperative Study of Perioperative Nutrition support. Presented at the 13th Clinical Congress of the American Society for Parenteral and Enteral Nutrition, February 4–8, 1989, Miami Florida.

44. Koretz R. Parenteral nutrition: is it oncologically logical? J Clin Oncol 1984;2:534–8.

45. McGeer AJ, Detsky AS, O'Rourke K. Parenteral nutrition in patients receiving cancer chemotherapy. Ann Int Med 1989;110:734.

46. Nirgiotis JD, Andrassy RJ. Bacterial translocation. In: Enteral nutrition (ed. Borlase BC, Bell SJ, Blackburn GL, Armour Forse R). New York: Chapman & Hall, 1994;37–46.

47. Bozzetti F, Amadori D, Bruera E et al. Report of the Consensus Meeting on Artificial Nutrition and Hydration in Terminal Cancer Patients. European Association of Palliative Care, Palermo, Italy, in press.

48. American College of Physicians. Position paper. Parenteral nutrition in patients receiving cancer chemotherapy. Ann Int Med 1989;110:734–6.

49. Weidorf SA, Lesne J, Wind D et al. Positive effect of prophylactic total parenteral nutrition on long term outcome of bone marrow transplantation. Transplantation 1987;43:833–8.

50. Szeluga DJ, Stuart RK, Brookmeyer R, Utermohlen V, Santos GW. Nutritional support of bone marrow recipients: a prospective randomized clinical trial comparing total parenteral nutrition to an enteral feeding program. Cancer Res 1987;47:3309–19.

51. Detsky AS, Baker JP, O'Rourke K, Goel V. Perioperative parenteral nutrition: a meta-analysis. Ann Int Med 1987;107:195–203.

52. Fan ST, Lo CM, Lai E, Chu KM, Liu CL Wong J. Perioperative nutritional support in patients undergoing hepatectomy for hepatocellular carcinoma. New Engl J Med 1994; 331(23):1547–52.

53. Twomey PL. Cost-effectiveness of total parenteral nutrition. In: Clinical nutrition: parenteral nutrition, 2nd edn. (ed. Rombeau JL, Caldwell MD. Philadelphia: Saunders, 1993;401–8.
54. Veterans Affairs Total Parenteral Nutrition Study Group. Perioperative total parenteral nutrition in surgical patients. New Engl J Med 1991;325(8):525–33.
55. Health and Public Policy Committee. Perioperative parenteral nutrition. Ann Int Med 1987;107:195–203.
56. Norton JA, Thom AK. Parenteral nutrition and the patient with cancer In: Clinical nutrition: parenteral nutrition, 2nd edn (ed. Rombeau JL, Caldwell MD). Philadelphia: Saunders, 1993;512–36.
57. Tchekmediyian NS, Halpert C, Ashley J, Heber D. Nutrition in advanced cancer: anorexia as an outcome variable and target to therapy. J Parent Ent Nutr 1993;16(6):88–92.
58. Tchekmedyian NS. Clinical approaches to nutritional support in cancer patient. Curr Opin Oncol 1993;5:633–8.
59. Daly JM, Lieberman MD, Goldfine J et al. Enteral nutrition with supplemental arginine, RNA and omega–3 fatty acids in postoperative patients: immunologic, metabolic and clinical outcomes. Surgery 1992;112:56–7.
60. Seifter E, Rittura G, Barbul A et al. Arginine: an essential amino-acid for injured rats. Surgery 1978;84:224–30.
61. Tachibama K, Mukai K Hiraoka I et al. Evaluation of the effect of arginine-enriched amino acid solution on tumor growth. J Parent Ent Nutr 1985;9:428.
62. Daly JM, Hoffman K, Lieberman M et al. Nutritional support in cancer patients. J Parent Ent Nutr 1990;14(5):244s–8s.
63. Chlebowosky RT, Heber D, Richardson B, Block JB. Influence of hydrazine sulphate on abnormal carbohydrate metabolism in cancer patients with weight loss. Cancer Res 1984;44:857–61.
64. Chlebowosky RT, Bulcavage L, Grosvenor et al. Hydrazine sulfate influence on nutritional status and survival in non small cell lung cancer. J Clin Oncol 1990;8:9.
65. Kosty M, Fleishman S, Herdon J et al. Cisplatin, vinblastine and hydrazine sulphate (NSC 150014) in advanced non small lung cancer: a randomized placebo-controlled, double-blind phase three study (Abstract 982). Pro Am Soc Clin Oncol 1992;11:294.
66. Gelin J, Moldawer LL, Lonroth C et al. Role of endogenous tumor necrosis factor alfa and interleukin–1 for experimental tumor growth and the development of cancer cachexia. Cancer Res 1991;51:415.
67. Sherry BA, Gelin J, Fong Y et al. Anticachectin/tumor necrosis factor alfa-antibodies attenuate development of cachexia in tumor models. FASEB J 1989;3:1956.
68. Schall TJ, Lewis M, Koller KJ et al. Molecular cloning and expression of a receptor for human tumor necrosis factor. Cell 1990;61:361–70.
69. McNamara M, Alexander R, Norton J. Cytokines and their role in the pathophysiology of cancer cachexia. J Parent Ent Nutr 1992;16:50s–5s.
70. Moley JF, Morrison SE, Norton JA. Insulin reversal of cancer cachexia in rats. Cancer Res 1985;45:4925–31.
71. Peacock JL, Norton JA. Impact of insulin on survival of cachectic tumor-bearing rats. J Parent Ent Nutr 1988;12:260–4.
72. Burt ME, Gorschboth CM, Brennan MF. A controlled, prospective, randomized trial evaluating the metabolic effects of enteral and parenteral nutrition in the cancer patients. Cancer 1982;49:1092–105.
73. Ward HC, Halliday D, Sim AJW. Protein and energy metabolism with biosynthetic human growth hormone. Ann Surgery 1987;206:56–61.

9

Pharmacological approach to cancer anorexia and cachexia

Robin Fainsinger

INTRODUCTION

Cachexia and anorexia are highly prevalent problems in advanced cancer patients. Anorexia refers to the loss of appetite and poor food intake, while cachexia refers to the weight loss suffered by these patients. Up to 80–90% of patients with advanced malignant disease have been reported to suffer from cachexia and anorexia (1, 2, see Chapter 6). The pathophysiology is complex and has been discussed in a previous chapter (Chapter 1).

While the ideal clinical management of cachexia and anorexia would be to remove the underlying disease, this is clearly not possible in the majority of advanced cancer patients.

Dietary counselling, enteral and parenteral nutrition, as well as management of associated chronic nausea of advanced cancer, have all been suggested as adjuvant therapies in the management of cachexia and anorexia. These aspects have been fully discussed in previous chapters (Chapters 2, 6, and 8). The high prevalence of cachexia and anorexia as well as the lack of results from the aforementioned therapies, has resulted in a variety of drugs being proposed and studied to assess their efficacy in treating the many patients with these devastating symptoms. This chapter will review the available information on corticosteroids, progestational drugs, cyproheptadine, hydrazine sulfate, cannabinoids, and pentoxifylline.

CORTICOSTEROIDS

It has been suggested that the increased sensation of well being associated with corticosteroid treatment, might alleviate some of the symptoms of advanced cancer patients, such as anorexia and asthenia (3, 4).

Moertel *et al.* (5) published a study of 116 patients with advanced gastrointestinal cancer, randomized to receive placebo or dexamethasone 0.75 mg or 1.5 mg orally four times daily. The patients receiving dexamethasone had significant symptomatic improvement in appetite and strength, although there was no antineoplastic effect, weight gain, or increased survival noted. The improvement disappeared after 4 weeks of treatment. Toxicity was reported to be low, with only one case of gastrointestinal hemorrhage.

Willcox *et al.* (6) reported a randomized, double-blind, cross-over trial of patients receiving 5 mg prednisolone three times daily. A significant improvement in appetite and well being was noted, although the majority of patients in the study were also receiving chemotherapy.

Bruera *et al.* (7) completed a randomized, double-blind, cross-over trial of oral methylprednisolone 16 mg twice a day. The patients received methylprednisolone or placebo for 5 days and after a 2-day wash-out period, patients were given the alternative treatment for a further 5 days. From day 13 all patients received 32 mg methylprednisolone daily for a further 20 days. At the end of the study, pain intensity and analgesic consumption had decreased significantly. In addition, appetite, food intake, and performance status were noted to have improved significantly. However, at the end of the 20-day open phase trial, all nutritional parameters had returned to the baseline level. Minimal toxicity associated with the methylprednisolone was noted during this study.

Two European multicenter studies used intravenous methylprednisolone to assess the effect of quality of life in patients with advanced cancer (8, 9). In the first study of 403 patients with pre-terminal cancer, 207 were treated with an 8-week course of 125 mg of methylprednisolone sodium succinate per day intravenously, while 196 received a placebo. A significant improvement in the quality of life was noted in the methylprednisolone group. for unexplained reasons, the female placebo-treated patients were noted to have a significantly lower mortality rate (8). In the second study (9), 173 female patients with terminal cancer were treated with either placebo or 125 mg of methylprednisolone sodium succinate intravenously daily for an 8-week period. The steroid-treated group were noted to have a significant improvement in quality of life for the duration of study. No differences were noted in the overall mortality rates or reported adverse effects between the treatment groups.

The mechanism of action of corticosteroids in patients with terminal cancer is not clear, although its euphoriant activity or the inhibition of prostaglandin metabolism may play a role. Despite the poor understanding of its mechanism of action as well as a paucity of controlled studies, the use of corticosteroids in a wide range of symptoms associated with advanced cancer has become widely accepted (10, 11).

In 1983 Hanks *et al.* (12) surveyed 373 patients admitted to a hospice over a 16-month period. Two hundred and eighteen (58%) patients received corticosteroids, with the most common reason being as a non-specific 'tonic'. Twenty-two out of 58 patients (38%) were reported to have responded to prednisolone, while seven out of 17 patients (41%) were said to have responded to dexamethasone. The incidence of side-effects was noted to be similar in both groups.

There are many side-effects noted with the use of corticosteroids in general and advanced cancer populations (12–15). Problems such as weakness, delirium, osteoporosis, and immunosuppression, are all commonly present in advanced cancer patients and might be exacerbated by corticosteroid treatment. For this reason some authors have advised caution in the use of steroids in advanced cancer patients (13, 14).

At present there is insufficient information on which corticosteroid to use, optimal dose, route of administration, or duration of therapy. In addition there are new steroids being developed that might prove to have therapeutic advantages in the future (16). The present evidence probably justifies a short trial of a corticosteroid in a symptomatic patient with advanced cancer who has no major contra-indication.

PROGESTATIONAL DRUGS

Clinical trials using progesterone derivatives in treating hormone responsive cancers, reported significant weight gain in patients showing tumor shrinkage as well as those showing no tumor response (17–20). As a result much research in recent years has focused on the use of megestrol acetate for the treatment of cachexia and anorexia in advanced cancer patients.

This research resulted in three randomized, double-blind, placebo-controlled trials to assess the effect of megestrol acetate on cachexia and anorexia in advanced cancer patients (21–23).

Bruera *et al.* (21) reported 40 consecutive patients with advanced hormone-insensitive tumors randomized to receive megestrol acetate (480 mg/day) or placebo for 7 days, followed by a cross-over to the other treatment at day 8 until day 15. None of the patients were receiving antineoplastic treatment. Assessments were made of appetite, pain, nausea, depression, energy, and well-being using a visual analog scale, as well as measurements of nutritional status, caloric intake, and side-effects. Patients choosing megestrol acetate over placebo or making no choice, were continued on megestrol acetate until they were unable to swallow or died. Megestrol acetate was assessed as being superior to placebo at 66 and 90% by the patient and investigator, respectively. Appetite, caloric intake, and nutritional status were noted to improve to a statistically significant degree. Side-effects were low with mild oedema and nausea reported in three and two patients, respectively.

Loprinzi *et al.* (22) studied 133 patients with documented cancer anorexia and cachexia who received megestrol acetate (800 mg/day) or placebo. Convincing evidence was provided that megestrol acetate stimulated appetite and food intake, with substantial weight gain observed in a number of patients. Eleven out of 67 patients on megestrol acetate gained 6.75 kg or more, as compared to only one out of 66 placebo-treated patients. Weight gain did not appear to be related to fluid accumulation, while in ten out of 11 patients weight gain did not appear to be related to a favorable tumor response.

Tchekmedyian *et al.* (23) reported 89 patients with hormone-insensitive tumors, treated with megestrol acetate (1600 mg/day) or placebo. Weight, anthropometric parameters, prealbumin, quality of life, appetite, and factors affecting food intake were assessed monthly. Analysis beyond 1 month was limited as only 53% of the patients could be assessed at 2 months. However, at the 1 month assessment, appetite had increased significantly more in patients receiving megestrol acetate, with patient-rated food intake also showing a larger increase than in the placebo-treated group. Prealbumin levels were noted to increase significantly more in patients receiving megestrol acetate.

Subsequent to these intial three studies there have been a number of other reports confirming the benefits of megestrol acetate in advanced cancer patients (24–27). Schmoll *et al.* (24) reported 55 patients with advanced cancer receiving only palliative therapy, who were randomized to receive either megestrol acetate at 480 or 960 mg/ day or placebo over an 8-week period. Of the 34 patients eligible for analysis, weight loss was seen in six out of eight patients in the placebo group as compared with five out of 15 patients in the low-dose megestrol acetate group and three out of 11 patients in the high-dose megestrol acetate group. Only one out of 11 patients in the placebo group gained weight, as compared to six out of 15 patients in the low-dose and six out of 11 patients in the high-dose megestrol acetate group. The median weight gains were 3 and 4 kg, respectively. Although there was a trend towards the beneficial effects of megestrol acetate, the small sample size precluded a demonstration of statistically significant differences. Side-effects were mild, with edema occurring in two patients, nausea and thrombosis in one patient, and sweating in one patient.

Heckmayr and Gatzeneier (25) reported 66 patients with advanced lung cancer given megestrol acetate for a 4–6 week period. Thirty-three patients received 160 mg/day and 33 patients received 480 mg /day. All antineoplastic treatments had been discontinued at least 4 weeks previously. Improved well-being and appetite was noted in 80% of patients, although the high-dose group showed an increase in mean weight gain of 3 kg as compared to the 2 kg of the low-dose group. The side-effect reported was peripheral edema in 5% of patients.

Feliu *et al.* (26) reported a study of 150 patients randomized to receive either megestrol acetate 240mg/day or placebo for a 2-month period. One hundred and twenty-eight patients were eligible for analysis. Twenty-one out of 66 patients treated with megestrol acetate experienced a weight gain of more than equal to 2 kg, while only five out of 62 given placebo experienced this gain (P < 0.01).

Splinter (27) reported 176 patients with advanced cancer given megestrol acetate 160mg three times per day after presenting with symptoms of anorexia. Fifty-seven patients (32%) reported an improvement in appetite and/or general well-being. The author concluded that as improvement is usually evident in 10 days and approximately 30% of patients in their experience will respond with minimal side-effects noted, it would seem worth while to proceed with a trial of megestrol acetate in anorectic patients.

Loprinzi *et al.* (28) noted that although many clinical trials have established that megestrol acetate causes appetite simulation and weight gain in advanced cancer patients with cachexia and anorexia, there is a lack of information to demonstrate the substance of the increased weight. They used dual-energy X-ray absorptiometry and tritiated body water methodologies, to perform body composition measurement in 12 patients with advanced breast cancer before receiving 800mg of oral megestrol acetate per day and thereafter at 2-month intervals. Four patients failed to gain weight, while the other eight patients gained a maximum of 2.1–16.5 kg over periods ranging from 5 weeks to 8 months. The results demonstrated that much of the weight gain was due to increased body fat stores, although increased hydration of fat-free mass suggested that subtle increases in extracellular fluid may have accounted for some of the weight gain. The main drawback of this trial would appear to be that none of the patients actually had the cachexia–anorexia syndrome, although the authors conclude there is good evidence to suggest that the results seen in this patient group would be applicable to other advanced cancer patients.

In a further study by Loprinzi *et al.* (29) the authors designed a trial to compare megestrol acetate doses ranging from 160 to 1280 mg per day. Three hundred and forty-two patients with cancer cachexia–anorexia syndrome were randomized to receive oral doses of megestrol acetate of 160, 480, 800, or 1280 mg/day with the study achieving a median follow-up duration of 66 days. No significant differences in study duration or survival were noted among the four treatment groups. Patients receiving 800 mg/day showed the greatest improvement in appetite and food intake, with a trend for more non-fluid weight gain in the patients receiving 800 or 1280 mg of megestrol acetate per day. There was no statistically significant difference in toxicities among the treatment groups. The authors felt that their data showed statistical confirmation that there was a positive dose–response effect from megestrol acetate on appetite and food intake, with the data suggesting that 800 mg/day was the most effective. However, due to the large number of tables and high cost of maintaining patients on 800 mg/day they felt it was probably reasonable to start patients on 160 mg /day and consider dose escalation only if no response was seen.

The mechanism of action of megestrol acetate remains poorly understood. As it is a steroidal hormone and corticosteroids have been noted to stimulate patient appetite, the question has been raised whether megestrol acetate is exerting its effect by acting as a corticosteroid. However, a megestrol acetate therapy is not known to result in side-effects noted with corticosteroid therapy, such as opportunistic infections, peptic ulcer disease, stria, myopathy, or cortisol depletion syndrome on drug withdrawal, this explanation seems unlikely (30).

Although most trials have reported low toxicity and good tolerance to megestrol acetate, several potential side-effects need to be considered. Experimental studies have shown that host weight gain with megestrol acetate treatment is associated with doubling of tumor weight (31). Other potential problems are impotence in sexually active males, vaginal spotting or bleeding in women, and thromboembolic complications. Although reported edema has usually been of a mild degree, patients with pre-existing edema or fluid overload problems could potentially be at increased risk for complications from this side-effect (32).

There have also been reports of megestrol acetate causing reversible suppression of the adrenal axis (33), diabetes mellitus in a patient with AIDS and cachexia (34), as well as a case report of a complex of symptoms that might have represented a megestrol acetate withdrawal syndrome following abrupt discontinuation of this drug (35).

CYPROHEPTADINE

Cyproheptadine is an antihistamine with antiserotonergic properties, better known for the treatment of allergies (36). There were some studies, mostly in the 1960s or early 1970s, that demonstrated that short-term administration of cyproheptadine could produce appetite- and weight-enchancing effects in non-cancer patients (37–39).

Kardinal *et al.* (40) reported a randomized, placebo-controlled, double-blind clinical trial, where 295 patients with advanced malignant disease received oral cyproheptadine 8 mg three times per day or placebo. The median treatment time was slightly over 1 month; however, only 25% of patients remained in the study for 3 months or more. Data suggested that although cyproheptadine appeared to stimulate patient appetite and food intake slightly, it did not significantly prevent progressive weight loss in this group of patients with advanced cancer cachexia.

It is worth noting that appetite stimulation was removed from the United States labeling of cyproheptadine approximately 20 years ago, with the clinical significance of the early studies showing appetite enhancement from cyproheptadine being criticized due to significant methodological defects (41). This has resulted in a recent decision in Canada to delete appetite stimulation as an indication for cyproheptadine use (42).

HYDRAZINE SULFATE

Hydrazine sulfate is an interesting drug that has been the subject of testing for approximately 30 years and has been found to have a variety of effects in man and experimental animals.

In 1970 Ray *et al*. (43) demonstrated that hydrazine sulfate inhibited gluconeogenesis in rats. More recently, Silverstine *et al*. (44) demonstrated that hydrazine sulfate may influence carbohydrate metabolism at the level of hepatic enzymes concerned with gluconeogenesis and glucose uptake in normal and cancerous rats, and in a further study (45) that pre-treatment with hydrazine sulfate significantly improved survival of mice challenged with salmonella enteritides endotoxin. *In vitro* experiments have demonstrated that hydrazine sulfate appeared to inhibit the activity of tumor necrosis factor, providing a hypothesis for a possible anticachexia effect (46).

Earlier results on hydrazine sulfate have been conflicting, with two uncontrolled trials (47, 48) suggesting possible useful benefits of hydrazine sulfate in advanced cancer patients, while three other clinical trials failed to confirm any beneficial effect (49–51).

Tayek *et al*. (52) reported a prospective double-blind trial in 12 cachectic patients with lung cancer, randomized to receive placebo or hydrazine sulfate 60 mg three times a day, for 30 days. Plasma lysine flux did not change significantly in the placebo group but did show a significant fall in the treated group, with serum albumin levels decreasing in the placebo group but remaining unchanged in the treatment group. The authors concluded that the administration of hydrazine sulfate may reduce amino acid flux and, thus, favorably influence metabolic abnormalities in patients with cancer cachexia.

Chlebowski *et al*. (53) recorded 24-hour dietary recall and body weight before and after 30 days of either placebo or hydrazine sulfate 60 mg three times a day in 101 cancer patients with weight loss. A total of 58 patients (57%) were evaluable. After 1 month, 83% of patients treated with hydrazine sulfate and only 53% of those on placebo maintained or increased their weight. Improvement of appetite was also noted more frequently in the group treated with hydrazine sulfate. Toxicity was mild, with 71% of patients reporting no toxic effects.

In a second trial by Chlebowski *et al*. (54) 65 patients with non-small cell lung cancer were randomly assigned to receive combination chemotherapy plus either placebo or hydrazine sulfate. Patients treated with hydrazine sulfate survived for a median of 292 days, compared to 187 days for those in the placebo group. Although this difference was not statistically significant, patients receiving hydrazine sulfate also showed a significant increase in caloric intake and serum albumin levels. This trial has been the subject of an editorial that focused on the hazards of small clinical trials and recommended cautious interpretation of the results until larger clinical trials have been completed (55).

In 1994 three large randomized, placebo controlled trials of hydrazine sulfate were reported by Loprinizi *et al.* (56, 57) and Kosty *et al.* (58). In the first study (56) 127 patients with metastatic colorectal cancer were randomized to receive hydrazine sulfate (60–180 mg/day) or placebo following a double-blind protocol. The results demonstrated trends both for poorer survival and quality of life in the hydrazine group. No significant diference was noted with regard to anorexia or weight loss. In the second study (57) 243 patients with a recent diagnosis of unresectable non-small cell lung cancer treated with cisplatin and etoposide, received hydrazine sulfate (60–180 mg/day) or placebo. Treatment response rates were similar: however, there was a trend to worse time to tumor progression and survival in the hydrazine sulfate group. No significant differences were noted in toxicity or quality of life. The authors concluded that both studies failed to demonstrate benefit to patients receiving hydrazine sulfate. Kosty *et al.* (58) reported on 266 advanced, non-small cell cancer patients receiving cisplatin-based combination chemotherapy, randomized to receive either hydrazine sulfate or placebo. This study also failed to demonstrate any benefit in the hydrazine sulfate group.

Herbert (59) commented that hydrazine sulfate has always been a 'questionable method' and with these three recent reports showing a failure of efficacy as well as safety, the fate of this drug as an ineffective treatment in cancer patients, should be sealed.

CANNABINOIDS

Appetite stimulation and weight gain are well-recognized effects with the use of marijuana and its derivatives (60). The active ingredient responsible for these effects is delta-nine-tetra-hydrocannabinol (THC) (61). Dronabinol and Marinol (in the United States) and Nabilone (in Canada) have been used as anti-emetics in cancer patients for some years, with many studies demonstrating the efficacy of THC in treating chemotherapy-induced nausea and vomiting (62–65). There have recently been some studies on the appetite-enhancement effects of THC in patients with advanced cancer.

Wadleigh *et al.* (66) conducted an open study in which patients with advanced cancer were treated with THC for up to 6 weeks, at doses of 2.5 mg/day (eight patients), 2.5 mg twice a day (nine patients) or 5 mg/day (13 patients). Five patients discontinued THC because of adverse effects, while three discontinued the drug because of progressive disease. In all groups patients continued to lose weight, although the rate of weight loss decreased with therapy in all doses. Symptomatic improvement was noted in both mood and appetite in the two higher dose groups.

Gorter (67) reported a retrospective analysis of ten male patients with cachexia associated with acquired immunodeficiency syndrome, treated with THC 2.5 mg three times per day, with the dosage adjusted depending on response and tolerance. During a 4–20 week study period, patients experienced a mean weight gain of 0.6 kg per month. Only two patients failed to gain weight while on THC. THC was reported to be well tolerated with minimal side-effects.

Nelson *et al.* (68) in a recent open study, gave THC to 19 advanced cancer patients with anorexia and a prognosis of > 4 weeks. Patients received THC 2.5 mg three times per day for 4 weeks. Eighteen patients were evaluable but only ten completed the entire 28-day study. Thirteen patients reported an improved appetite, however ten rated this as 'slight improvement'. The authors noted the need for controlled studies to determine better the efficacy and usefulness of THC in this patient population.

PENTOXIFYLLINE

Pentoxifylline is a substituted methylxanthine that is approved for the treatment of intermittent claudication. It has recently been suggested that it might have a role in the cachexia–anorexia syndrome as it has been shown to decrease tumor necrosis factor (TNF) activity *in vitro* and *in vivo*. Pentoxifylline had been shown to lower TNF both in endotoxin-treated normal human volunteers (69), as well as in similarly treated rodents (70, 71).

In 1990, Dezube *et al.* (72) reported a patient with advanced lung cancer given two 1-week courses of oral pentoxifylline 400 mg three times a day. Both courses of therapy resulted in increased well-being, appetite, and ability to perform activities of daily living. More recently Dezube *et al.* (73) have reported further results on the effect of pentoxifylline on TNF. TNF–actin ratios were determined in peripheral blood mononuclear cells isolated from eight healthy volunteers. TNF-actin ratios were then determined in 15 cancer patients, eight of whom had ratios significantly higher ($P < 0.05$) than those in the normal volunteers. Seven patients were then treated on eight occasions with pentoxifylline 400 mg every 8 hours. Four patients were treated for 1 week, two for 3 weeks, and one was cycled through the drug twice. On all three occasions, when the initial TNF-actin ratios were greater than the normal range determined in healthy volunteers, pentoxifylline suppressed these ratios dramatically within one week of treatment. On the five occasions when TNF-actin ratios did not differ significantly from the normal volunteers, pentoxifylline did not lower the ratios to subnormal values. Due to the limited sample size, formal assessment of quality of life was not performed. However, of the seven patients, four reported an increased sense of comfort and well-being, as well as improved appetite and ability to perform activities of daily living. However, a larger study with randomized double-blind placebo-controlled design and more sophisticated quality of life assessments, is needed to confirm that pentoxifylline can indeed improve appetite and well-being.

EICOSAPENTAENOIC ACID (EPA)

The polyunsaturated fatty acid EPA has been shown to inhibit the action of tumor-produced, lipid-mobilizing factor in an *in vivo* assay and to inhibit the development of cachexia in an *in vivo* model (74). In addition to preserving adipose tissue, EPA has also been reported to prevent loss of skeletal muscle by a large reduction in the rate of protein degradation (75). Further clinical studies are required to determine the efficacy of EPA in advanced cancer patients with cachexia.

CLINICAL GUIDELINES

The management of cachexia in advanced cancer patients should first attempt to maximize oral intake by allowing the patient flexibility in type, quantity, and timing of meals. The advice of a dietitian should be requested where possible (see Chapter 7). Adequate management of associated nausea must also be achieved as a necessary initial step.

In those patients in whom profound anorexia persists as the main problem, pharmacological management might be appropriate. The decision-making process will have to take into account the patient's overall prognosis, adequacy of control of other symptoms, for example pain, the extent to which the patient views the cachexia and anorexia as a problem, and, finally, the affordability of the proposed pharmacological management given the patient's economic circumstances. Economic considerations vary widely with the different treatment options (Table 9.1) and some of the suggested therapies can be costly. The cost of therapy may vary widely in different countries, with therapeutic decisions tailored accordingly.

Table 9.1 Medical treatments for cancer cachexia

	Daily dose	Cost per day (Canadian funds) 1994 prices
Megesterol acetate	160 mg	5.49
Dexamethasone	4 mg	0.14
Pentoxifylline	400 mg three times daily	1.07
Cyproheptadine	8 mg three times daily	1.07
Nabilone	1 mg twice daily	13.94
Dronabinol	Not available in Canada	
Hydrazine sulfate	Not available as commercial preparation	

Megestrol acetate is the therapy receiving the most attention and research at present and would certainly appear to have positive benefits for many advanced cancer patients, particularly those expected to survive for weeks to months. It would seem reasonable to start with 160 mg/day and titrate the dose upwards according to patient response.

Corticosteroids would appear to be useful, particularly in patients with a shorter expected survival, due to a short-lasting effect. In addition, the relatively low cost might make it an attractive option for some patients. A commonly recommended starting dose would be dexamethasone 4 mg/day, with dose titration and treatment duration based on response and overall prognosis.

Hydrazine sulfate has been increasingly studied in recent years and the negative results in well-designed studies would appear to indicate that there is no basis for recommending this drug for cancer patients with anorexia and/or cachexia.

The remaining suggested treatments have received insufficient evaluation to date to be recommended as any more than second line treatments and could be used in individual patients in a carefully monitored therapeutic trial or as part of a randomized, controlled study (see Future research guidelines below).

Cyproheptadine is relatively easily available for a therapeutic trial, but early studies in non-cancer patients have been criticized and it has been infrequently reported in recent years.

Cannabinoids are the most expensive of the treatment options, but have been reported to be effective in some patients in small uncontrolled studies.

Pentoxifylline is readily available and, although the data is preliminary, it is reasonably inexpensive and a therapeutic trial might be justified in some patients.

FUTURE RESEARCH

There are presently placebo-controlled, double-blind, clinical trials which have shown appetite stimulation for both corticosteroids and progestational drugs in patients with cancer anorexia–cachexia syndrome. Future trials are required to compare more definitively progestational drugs versus corticosteroids for appetite stimulation and weight gain in advanced cancer patients.

Other suggested treatments, such as cannabinoids and pentoxifylline, require further evaluation and publication of well-designed studies before being generally recommended for use in advanced cancer patients with cachexia and anorexia.

Improved knowledge of the pathophysiology of cancer and AIDS-induced cachexia would assist in the development of more effective treatments and might provide a new locus for therapeutic intervention. Better understanding of the metabolic changes associated with cachexia, might enable the development of drugs or 'designer' diets containing different proportions of amino acids or fatty acids.

Finally, it is not enough to demonstrate in advanced cancer patients that certain drugs are able to stimulate appetite, increase caloric intake, and cause a temporary improvement in nutritional status. In this patient group it is perhaps more important to show that patients achieve symptomatic benefit and an improved life quality that outweighs the potential side-effects and economic costs of the treatment.

REFERENCES

1. Grant JP. Preventing complications of surgery: emphasis on nutrtional factors. In Physicians' guide to cancer care complications: prevention and management (ed. Laszlo J, Dakken N). New York, NY: Dekker, 1986; 48–52.
2. Bruera E, MacDonald RN. Nutrition in cancer patients: an update and review of our experience. J Pain Symptom Manage 1988;3:133–40.
3. Schell H. Adrenal corticosteroid therapy in far-advanced cancer. Geriatrics 1972;27:131–41.
4. Twycross RG. Continuing in terminal care: an overview in advances in pain research and therapy. In: Proceedings of the International Symposium of Pain of Advanced Cancer, Vol 2 (ed. Bonica J, Ventafridda V). New York: Raven Press, 1979;617–34.
5. Moertel C, Schutt AG, Reiteneier RJ, Hahn RG. Corticosteroid therapy of pre-terminal gastrointestinal cancer. Cancer 1974;33:1607–9.
6. Willcox J, Corr J, Shaw J et al. Prednisolone as an appetite stimulant in patients with cancer. BMJ 1984;200:37.

7. Bruera E, Roca E, Cedaro L, Carraro S, Chacon R. Action of oral methylprednisolone in terminal cancer patients: a prospective randomized double-blind study. Cancer Treat Rep 1985;69:751–54.

8. Robustelli Della Cuna G, Pellegrini A, Piazzi M. Effect of methylprednisolone sodium succinate on quality of life in pre-terminal cancer patients: a placebo controlled multi-center study. Eur J of Cancer Clin Oncol 1989;25:1817–21.

9. Popiela, T, Lucchi R, Giongo F. Methylprednisolone as palliative therapy for female terminal cancer patients. Eur J Cancer Clin Oncol 1989;25:1823–9.

10. Ettinger AB, Portenoy RK. The use of corticosteroids in the treatment of symptoms associated with cancer. J Pain Symptom Manage 1988;3:99–103.

11. Far WC. The use of corticosteroids for symptom management in terminally ill patients. Am J Hospice Care 1990;1:41–6.

12. Hanks GW, Trueman T, Twycross RG. Corticosteroids in terminal cancer—a prospective analysis of current practice. Postgrad Med J 1983;59:702–6.

13. Needham PR, Daley AG, Lennard RF. Steroids in advanced cancer: survey of current practice. BMJ 1992;305:999.

14. Twycross RG. Corticosteroids in advanced cancer. BMJ 1992;305:969–70.

15. MacDonald SM, Hagen N, Bruera E. Proximal weakness in a patient with hepatocellular carcinoma. J Pain Symptom Manage 1994;9(5):346–50.

16. Williams CN. New steroids. Can J Gastroenterol 1993;7:588.

17. Cavalli F, Goldhirsch A, Young IF. Randomized trial of low vs. high dose medroxypro-gesterone acetate in the treatment of postmenopausal patients with advanced breast cancer In: Role of medroxyprogesterone in endocrine-related tumors (ed. Pellegrini A, Robustelli G). New York: Raven Press, 1983; 69–76.

18. Tchekmedyian S, Tait N, Moody M et al. High dose megestrol acetate; a possible treatment for cachexia. J Am Med Assoc 1987;257:1195–99.

19. Tchekmedyian S, Tait N, Moody M et al. Appetite stimulation with megestrol acetate in cachectic cancer patients. Seminars Oncol 1986;13:37–43.

20. Cruz JM, Muss HB, Brockschmidt JK et al. Weight changes in woman with metastatic breast cancer treated with megestrol acetate: a comparison of standard vs a high dose therapy. Seminars Oncol 1990;17 (Suppl); 63–7.

21. Bruera E, Macmillan K, Hanson J, Kuehn N, MacDonald RN. A controlled trial of megestrol acetate on appetite, caloric intake, nutritional status, and other symptoms in patients with advanced cancer. Cancer 1990;66:1279–82.

22. Loprinzi CL, Ellison NM, Schaid DJ et al. Controlled trial of megestrol acetate for the treatment of cancer, anorexia and cachexia. J Natl Cancer Inst 1990;82:1127–32.

23. Tchekmedyian S, Hakman M, Siau J et al. Megestrol acetate in cancer anorexia and weight loss. Cancer 1992;69:1268–74.

24. Schmoll E, Wilke H, Thole R. Megestrol acetate in cancer cachexia. Seminars Oncol 1991;1(Suppl 2):32–4.

25. Heckmayr M, Gatzeneier U. Treatment of cancer weight loss in patients with advanced lung cancer. Oncology 1992;49 (Suppl 2):32–4.

26. Feliu J, Gonzalez–Baron M, Berrocal A. Usefulness of megestrol acetate in cancer cachexia and anorexia. Am J Clin oncol 192;15:436–40.

27. Splinter TA. Cachexia and cancer: a clinicians view. Anna Oncol 1992;3(Suppl 3):25–7.

28. Loprinzi CL, Schaid DJ, Dose AN et al. Body-composition changes in patients who gain weight while receiving megestrol acetate. J Clin Oncol 1993;11:152–4.

29. Loprinzi CL, Michalak JC, Schaid DJ. Phase three evaluation of four doses of megestrol acetate as therapy for patients with cancer anorexia and/or cachexia. J Clin Oncol 1993;11:762–7.

30. Lopriniz CL, Goldberg RM, Burnham NL. Cancer-associated anorexia and cachexia. Drugs 1992;43:499–506.

31. Beck SA, Tisdale MJ. Effect of megestrol acetate on weight loss induced by tumor narcosis

factor "alpha" and a cachexia inducing tumor (MAC16) in NMRI mice. Br J Cancer 1990;62:420–4.

32. Tchekmedyian NS. Clinical approaches to nutritional support in cancer. Curr Opin Oncol 1993;5:633–8.

33. Loprinzi CL, Jensen MD, Jiang N et al. Effect of megestrol acetate on the human pituitary–adrenal axis. Mayr Clin Proc 1992;67:1160–2.

34. Henry K, Rathgaber S, Sullivan C et al. Diabetes mellitus induced by megestrol acetate in a patient with AIDS and cachexia. Ann Med 1992;116:53–4.

35. Nathwani D, Green S, Heslop J et al. Beneficial response to megestrol acetate in AIDS related cachexia and a possible megestrol withdrawal-associated syndrome? Acta Derm Venereol 1990;70:520–1.

36. Munroe. I Cyproheptadine (editorial) Lancet 1978;1:367–8.

37. Shah N. A double-blind study on appetite stimulation and weight gain with cyproheptadine adjunct to specific therapy in pulmonary tuberculosis. Curr Med Pract 1968;12:861–4.

38. Noble RE. Effect of cyproheptadine on appetite and weight gain in adults. J Am Med Assoc 1969;209:2054–5.

39. Pawlowski G. Cyproheptadine: weight gain and appetite stimulation in essential anorexic adults. Curr Ther Res 1975;18:673–8.

40. Kardinal C, Loprinzi CL, Schaid DJ et al. A controlled trial of cyproheptadine in cancer patients with anorexia and/or cachexia. Cancer 1990;65:2657–62.

41. Lexchin J. Appetite stimulant claim deleted from label. Can Family Physician 1994;40:20–22.

42. Durbin RL. Response. Can Family Physician 1994;40:22.

43. Ray BD, Hanson RL, Lardy HA. Inhibition by hydrazine of gluconeogenesis in the rat. J Bio chem 1970;5:690–6.

44. Silverstein R, Bhatia P, Svoboda DS. Effect of hydrazine sulfate on glucose-regulating enzymes in the normal and cancerous rat. Immunopharmacology 1989;17:37–43.

45. Silverstein R, Christofferson CA, Morrison DC. Modulation of endotoxin lethality in mice hydrazine sulfate. Infect Immun 1989;57:2072–8.

46. Hughes TK, Cadet P, Larnad CS. Modulation of tumor necrosis factor activities by potential anticachexia compound hydrazine sulfate. Int J Immunopharmacol 1989;11:501–5.

47. Gold J. Use of hydrazine sulfate in terminal and pre terminal cancer patients: results of investigation of new drug study in 84 evaluable patients. Oncology 975;32:1–10.

48. Gershanovich ML, Danova LA, Ivin BA et al. Results of clinical study of antitumor action of hydrazine sulfate. Nutr Cancer 1981;3:7–12.

49. Spremulli E, Wampler GL, Regelson W. Clinical study of hydrazine sulfate in advanced cancer patients. Cancer Chemother Pharmacol 1979;3:121–4.

50. Lener HJ, Regelson W. Clinical trial of hydrazine sulfate in solid tumors. Cancer Treat Rep 1976;60:959–60.

51. Ocho AM, Wittes RE, Krakoff RH. Trial of hydrazine sulfate (NSC-150014) in patients with cancer. Cancer Chemother Rep 1975;59:1151–4.

52. Tayek JA, Heber D, Chlebowski RT. Effect of hydrazine sulfate on whole body protein breakdown measured by C-lysine metabolism in lung cancer patients. Lancet 1987;2:241–4.

53. Chelebowski RT, Bulcavate L, Grosvenor M et al. Hydrazine sulfate in cancer patients with weight loss: a placebo controlled clinical experience. Casncer 1987;59:406–10.

54. Chlebowski RT, Bulcavate L, Grosvenor M et al. Hydrazine sulfate influence on nutritional status and survival in non small cell lung cancer. J Clin Oncol 1990;8:9–15.

55. Piantadosi S. Hazards of small clinical trails. J Clin Oncol 1990;8:1–3.

56. Loprinzi CL, Kuross SA, O'Fallon JR et al. Randomized placebo-controlled evaluation on hydrazine sulfate in patients with advanced colorectal cancer. J Clin Oncol 1994;12:1121–5.

57. Loprinzi CL, Goldberg RM, Su JQ. Placebo-controlled trial of hydrazine sulfate in patients with newly diagnosed non-small-cell lung cancer. J Clin Oncol 1994;12:1126–9.

58. Kosty MP, Fleishman SB, Herndon JE et al. Cisplatin, vinblastine, and hydrazine sulfate in advanced non-small-cell lung cancer; a randomized placebo-controlled, double-blind phase III study of the cancer and leukemia group B. J Clin Oncol 1994;12:1113–20.

59. Herbert V. Three stakes in hydrazine sulfate's heart, but questionable cancer remedies, like vampires, always rise again. J Clin Oncol 1994;12:1107–8.

60. Foltin RW, Fischman MW, Byrne MF. Effects of smoked marijuana on food intake and body weight of humans living in a residential laboratory. Appetite 1988;11:1–14.

61. Mechoulam R, McCallum NK, Lander V et al. Aspects of cannabis chemistry and metabolism. In: The pharmacology of marijuana (ed. Braude MC, Szara S). New York, NY: Raven Press, 1976:39–48.

62. Frytak S, Moertel CJ, O'Fallon JR et al. Delta-nine-tetrahydrocannabinol as an antiemetic for patients receiving cancer chemotherapy. Ann Int Med 1979;91:825–30.

63. Lucas VS, Laszio J. Delta-nine-tetrahydrocannabinol for refractory vomiting induced by cancer chemotherapy. JAMA 1980;243:1241–3.

64. Underleeider JT, Andrysiak T, Fairbanks L et al. Cannabis in cancer chemotherapy. Cancer 1992;50:636–5.

65. Lane M, Vogel CL, Ferguson J et al. Dronabinol and prochlorperazine in combination for treatment of cancer chemotherapy-induced nausea and vomiting. J Pain Symptom Manage 991;6:352–9.

66. Wadleigh R, Spaulding M, Lembersky B et al. Dronabinol enhancement of appetite and cancer patients. Proc Am Soc Oncol 1990;9:331.

67. Gorter R. Management of anorexia–cachexia associated with cancer and HIV infection. Oncology 1991;5 (Suppl 9):13–17.

68. Nelson K, Walsh D, Deeter P et al. A phase II study of delta-nine-tetrahydrocannabinol for appetite stimulation in cancer-associated anorexia. J Palliat Care 1994;10:14–18.

69. Zabel P, Schonharting MM, Wolter DT et al. Oxpentifylline in endotoxaemia. Lancet 1989:1474–77.

70. Noel P, Nelson S, Bokullic R et al. Pentoxifylline inhibits lipopolysaccharide-induced serum tumor necrosis factor and mortality. Life Signs 1990;47:1023–9.

71. Schade UF. Pentoxifylline increases survival in murin endotoxin shock and decreases formation of tumor necrosis factor. Circ Shock 190;31:171–81.

72. Dezube BJ, Fridovich-Keil JL, Bouvard I et al. Pentoxifylline and wellbeing in patients with cancer. Lancet 1990;335:662.

73. Dezube BJ, Sherman ML, Friadovich-Keil JL, Down-regulation of tumor necrosis factor expression by pentoxifylline in cancer patients: a pilot study. Cancer Immunother 1993;36:57–60.

74. Tisdale MJ, Beck SA. Inhibition of tumor-induced lipolysis *in vitro* and cachexia and tumor growth *in vivo* by eicosapentaenoic acid. Biochem Pharmacol 1991;41:103–7.

75. Beck SA, Smith KS, Tisdale MJ. Anticachexic and anti tumor effect of eicosapentaenoic acid and its effect on protein turnover. Cancer Res 1991;51:6089–93.

10

Methods for artificial feeding and drainage of the gastrointestinal tract

Carla Ripamonti and Brett T. Gemlo

INTRODUCTION

Cancer patients have the highest incidence of malnutrition in hospitalized populations (1).

Cancer-induced malnutrition has been found to be present in more than two-thirds of patients with advanced and terminal disease (2, 3) and 4.4–23% of cancer patients die mainly from cachexia (4–6).

Of the 3047 patients who were included in different studies of the Eastern Cooperative Oncology Group, weight loss was in the range of 31–40% in patients with non-Hodgkin's lymphomas, breast cancer, acute non-lymphocytic leukemia, and sarcomas. The incidence of weight loss was in the range of 48–61% in patients with unfavorable non-Hodgkin's lymphoma, colonic cancer, prostatic, and lung cancer and 83–87% in patients with pancreatic or gastric cancer (7).

Different authors have shown that patients with upper gastrointestinal cancers and in particular cancer of the esophagus are more frequently affected with malnutrition (8–10).

The most frequent causes of malnutrition are summarized in Table 10.1 and are due to a combination of metabolic abnormalities, endogenous peptides, malabsorption, and decreased food intake (11–18). Anorexia and swallowing-associated difficulties due to neurological or malignant causes are the two primary indications for artificial feeding.

Table 10.2 shows the most frequent causes of dysphagia.

Anorexia is one of the most frequent symptoms in cancer patients with a prevalence ranging from 31 (19) to 85% (20) but the causes are not well understood (21).

Over the last 20 years there has been great progress regarding total parenteral nutrition (TPN) and enteral artificial nutrition (EN) (22) for patients who cannot take food by mouth or cannot swallow, or in order to set up controlled feeding in anorexic patients.

When the gastrointestinal tract s functional, enteral feeding is preferable to TPN because it is more physiological, easier and safer to manage, of lower cost, and can be performed easily at home by most patients. EN may prevent gut mucosal atrophy and preserve gastrointestinal immune function (23). Furthermore, TPN has proved not to give any significant advantage in comparison to EN in patients with functional bowels (24–26).

Table 10.1 Causes of malnutrition in patients with advanced cancer

Decreased intake	Malabsorption	Increased consumption
Anorexia	Bowel obstruction	By tumor
Dysphagia	Jaundice	Metabolism
Odynophagia	Pancreatic tumors	Abnormal metabolisms
Taste alterations	Radiotherapy	Tumor-related substances
Oral cavity lesions	Chemotherapy	
Dry mouth	Crohn's disease	
Early satiety	Fistulas	
Nausea/vomiting	Short-bowel syndrome	
Delayed gastric emptying		
Food aversion		
Tumor-released substances		
Depression		
Wish to die		
Cognitive failure		
Hospitalization		

This chapter considers the role of enteral tubes, gastrostomy, and jejunostomy for feeding and venting purposes in advanced cancer patients. Colostomy and rectal intubation for decompressive procedures will also be examined. Even if, at least for a limited time, artificial feeding (TPN or EN) can prevent further nutritional deterioration, its role in cancer cachexia is still controversial; in addition to simple starvation, many patients present metabolic changes similar to those seen during infection and will not respond positively to even aggressive nutritional support (11).

Table 10.2 Causes of dysphagia

Obstructive
    Cancer in the mouth, pharynx, and esophagus
    Tumoral infiltration of the pharyngo-oesophageal wall
    Extrinsic compression due to mediastinic mass
Neurological
    Perineuronal tumor spread (vagus, sympathicus)
    Paralysis of the lower cranial nerves
    Esophageal spasms
    Strokes, Parkinson's disease, Alzheimer's disease, motor neurone disease, multiple sclerosis, muscle disease
Iatrogenic
    Demolishing surgical intervention in the mouth
    Post-RT fibrosis in the head and neck area
    Osteoradionecrosis of the mandible
    Fistulas
    Candidiasis

Many controversies about artificial feeding also stem from the fact that cancer patients eligible to receive enteral feeding are frequently different from one another with regard to life expectancy, performance status, quality of life, and suitability for a proper oncologic or palliative treatment of their symptoms. Artificial feeding in advanced cancer patients with no possibility of specific oncologic therapy is still an open and debatable issue in a palliative care setting. In our opinion, no kind of artificial feeding can be considered for terminal cancer patients who present prognostic indicators of impending death (27, 28); hydration should be taken into consideration for these patients, if required (29, 30) (see Chapter 8). However, for patients having a life expectancy of a few months, artificial feeding may be indicated.

Artificial feeding for advanced cancer patients should not have the simple aim of prolonging life but also, and above all, improving quality of life and performance status thus preventing further rapid weight loss and malnutrition. The effect of enteral nutrition on quality of life is difficult to assess because possible benefits from nutrition can be hidden by the progression of the disease. Nelson *et al.* (31) studied 53 patients (mainly with cancer and progressive neurological disease) of which 50% reported that their quality of life was improved by home EN, 39% reported that their life quality was maintained, and in the remaining patients the quality of life had deteriorated due to discomfort caused by EN.

With a patient suffering from symptoms that could be managed by enteral feeding, the aims of nutritional support should be established before the onset of treatment and then evaluated if appropriate for each patient in terms of comfort/discomfort, their expectations, and morbidity due to the different techniques employed.

Some of the possible aims of enteral alimentation in advanced cancer patients are as follows:

1. Feeding patients that are not able to swallow but are hungry.

2. Stabilizing the nutritional state to avoid a rapid and progressive worsening or a drastic change in the body image that could bring about depression and desperation.

3. Minimizing progressive physical weakness due to malnutrition that could determine feelings of helplessness and, thus, loss of self-esteem.

4. Satisfying the expectations of the patients who consider anorexia and the inability to eat as synonymous of death and who believe that feeding means survival.

5. Feeding of patients suffering from intestinal malignant partial obstruction which is aggravated by the ingestion of solid food. For these patients continuous infusion of a liquid enteral diet can be of benefit in reducing symptoms.

6. Feeding the patient whose weight loss is exacerbated due to complications such as fistulas, short bowel obstruction, vomiting, or malabsorption induced by the tumor itself or the treatment (32).

After having established the desired aim, it would be necessary to verify whether EN is practicable and suitable. The following questions should be answered before beginning nutritional support.

1. What would change for the patient if cachexia were reversed or the progressive wasting prevented?

2. Is EN indicated in the case of the patient's clinical situation?

3. Is the clinical status of the patient sufficiently stable to begin EN?

4. Is this form of nutrition technically possible?

5. Is it better to feed the patient by enteral tube, gastrostomy, or jejunostomy?

6. Is EN also accepted by the patient from a psychological point of view?

7. Will the patient (and/or relatives) consent to this form of therapy?

8. Will the patient live long enough to benefit from artificial nutrition (at least 2–3 months)?

9. Will the patient live better than before treatment?

10. Will the patient have the possibility to go home and continue treatment there?

11. Will the patient have care givers who can manage EN at home?

12. Does the patient present other physical and/or psychological symptoms that are difficult to manage?

13. Is the patient likely to die of multiple metastatic involvement of vital organs before food deprivation?

14. Is EN feasible in terms of costs and benefits?

After having take the decision to begin EN, the patient and family members must be trained for home management of EN (33). The type of enteral feeding products to be used, the quantity, and the frequency (continuously or by cyclic nocturnal administration) which can vary in relation to the patient's age and clinical condition and the energy density of the feeding need to be decided.

Complications may arise if the rate of administration into the small bowel is inadvertently increased and diarrhea is more likely to occur than if the feed is introduced into the stomach. The use of a pump may help prevent this complication in jejunostomy feeding. With gastrostomy feeding a pump may also help prevent gastric pooling which can lead to regurgitation, vomiting, and aspiration pneumonia. Furthermore, it should be noted that pharmacological interaction may occur between the drugs and the nutritional products (Table 10.3) (34–36).

Table 10.3 Interactions of enteral products and drugs

---

1. Syrups containing iron mixed with enteral products may cause gelling and rapid coagulation. Pulverized preparations overcome this problem.
2. Lanoxin elixirs when mixed with enteral feed and is kept at room temperature for 24 hours, causing coagulation.
3. Phenytoin absorption can be reduced until 70% if it is administered during feed infusion. Stopping the feed to administer the drug avoids the problem.

References: (34–36)

FEEDING METHODS

Nasoenteral tube

Enteral tubes introduced through the nose transit the pharynx and reach the stomach, duodenum, or jejunum. These tubes have been used for EN administration in patients unable to swallow for a long time now. They can be useful in the short-term but often prove to be rigid and badly tolerated, because over a long period of time many complications may arise (Table 10.4) making it inadvisable for a period over 2–3 weeks. The correct positioning of the tube is verified radiographically. In order to avoid stagnation of the tube feed which could produce bacterial overgrowth the tube should have lateral holes at the very tip.

Table 10.4 Complications of nasoenteric intubation

Discomfort for the patient
Psychological distress
Tube misplacement
Frequent spontaneous expulsions
Spontaneous migration of the tip of the tube
Nasal or pharyngeal irritation
Impair the function of the GE sphincter causing or exacerbating esophageal reflux
Esophagitis
Esophageal perforation, bleeding, strictures
Aspiration pneumonia
Pulmonary intubation

Nowadays, soft, small-diameter (silastic) enteral tubes are used; their tips are weighted with mercury and are well tolerated with a low risk of spontaneous expulsion and are more indicated for EN.

However, different authors (37–39) contest the use of these tubes because of the high cost. According to Pichard (37), fixation of the tube plays a critical role in EN. If it is poorly secured it may move during swallowing or activity giving rise to nausea and epithelial lesions. The rate of spontaneous expulsion of the tube is very high: approximately 23% within 24 hours of starting feeding (40) and in two-thirds of elderly patients are expelled (41). In general, the tube should be fixed to the side of the nose then to the hair line above the ear. In patients with esophageal cancer an enteral tube should be used for patients with short life expectancy when an esophageal prothesis is not indicated or in the case where they already have a prothesis which is obstructed.

For enteral feeding administration it is advisable to use an infusion pump which allows continuous 24-hour infusion, thus reducing digestive side-effects (such as rapid gastric distension) caused by a rapid intake of hyperosmolar solutions. Although tube feeding may be a necessary medical procedure, its psychological impact should be taken into consideration, in particular when enteral tube feeding has to be administered for prolonged periods, as the tube can interfere with social rehabilitation.

As a contemporary surgeon said, 'It is more important for a surgeon to carry a nasogastric tube than a stethoscope in his pocket'.

Patients have always reported that nasogastric intubation creates discomfort and they would rather vomit two to three times a day than have the tube. Notwithstanding this fact, gastric decompression via this method has gained widespread acceptance and for years the disadvantages or complications were not taken into consideration. Only now are we beginning to realize that the role of nasoenteric intubation should be used only in particular cases (Table 10.5).

Table 10.5 Indications for nasoenteric intubation

When the feeding period is likely to be short (no more than 2–3 weeks).
Acute gastric dilatation.
Management of vomiting due to duodenal occlusion when a venting percutaneous endoscopic gastrostomy is not performable.

The nasogastric tube is usually employed post-operatively with the aim of decompression of the abdomen to prevent complications such as vomiting, gas and fluid distension, and wound dehiscence. As often happens in medical practice, the procedure has remained unquestioned for a long time despite the discomfort it causes the patient.

It is well known that the majority of the secretions of the digestive tract are reabsorbed along the intestinal tract and, furthermore, that the distress caused by the tube can increase the volume of air swallowed. A recent prospective randomized controlled clinical trial was carried out to evaluate the usefulness of gastric decompression intubation after digestive tract surgery in 109 patients divided into two groups with and without tubes (42). The results show that abdominal distension, pyrosis, sour stomach, otalgia, dysphagia, odynophagia, and atelectasis occurred significantly more often in intubated patients. No significant differences were found between the two groups in the duration of hospitalization, regarding the time to begin peroral fluid intake, occurrence of hiccups, vomiting, nausea, parotiditis, nasal septum necrosis, anastomotic leak, and wound dehiscence. Thus, routine post-operative use of a nasogastric tube is not recommended, but should be used selectively in the treatment of post-operative acute gastric dilation or in the presence of frequent vomiting caused by delayed gastric emptying.

In patients with inoperable bowel obstruction, the usual hospital treatment used for controlling vomiting, pain, and abdominal distension is nasogastric suction and liquid supplementation. This is useful for decompression of the stomach or intestine and for correcting fluid and electrolyte imbalance before surgery or while awaiting a decision regarding alternative treatment. A review of the surgical literature shows that only up to 14% of patients with malignant obstruction respond to conservative treatment (43). The tube often becomes occluded and requires flushing or replacement. During long-term drainage, a nasogastric tube can interfere with coughing to clear pulmonary secretions and may be associated with nasal cartilage erosion, otitis media, aspiration pneumonia, esophagitis, and bleeding (44).

Prolonged nasogastric suction and intravenous fluids for symptomatic treatment of inoperable patients is not recommended. This treatment involves hospitalization, immobility, and can create discomfort in patients who are already distressed by previous anticancer and surgical therapies.

At present, symptoms caused by inoperable gastrointestinal obstruction can be managed in 80% of the cases through adequate pharmacological therapy (45). A nasogastric intubation should only be considered when pharmacological therapy for symptom control is ineffective and when it is impossible to perform a venting percutaneous gastrostomy in patients with complete malignant bowel obstruction. In this case decompression by means of tubes can be carried out once a day or every 2 days, thus avoiding a permanent nasogastric tube.

Gastrostomy

Traditionally, the most versatile and efficient method of decompression of the gastrointestinal (GI) tract has been gastrostomy. Its proximal anatomic position makes it more durable if intra-abdominal conditions change and more proximal sites of obstruction develop and its high position in the GI tract makes feeding more efficient if obstruction is not present.

Gastric decompression obviates the need for nasogastric intubation, except in cases of high-grade esophageal obstruction. It is also very useful for patients with extensive head and neck cancers, allowing maintenance of enteral nutrition (46). This provides a significant increase in quality of life in patients with malignant bowel obstruction, eliminating tube discomfort, facial disfigurement, lack of mobility, and enables the obstructed patient oral intake without vomiting (47). It also reduces pulmonary complications and the risk of gastroesophageal reflux secondary to obturation of the esophageal sphincter. In non-obstructed patients it allows feeding regimens which are easy to administer and do not always require continuous administration pump systems.

Current options in the use of gastrostomy tubes primarily revolve around the method of insertion of the tube. There is little role for 'blow hole' or gastrocutaneous fistulae which are not controlled by a tube because of the corrosive nature of gastric secretions. Tube gastrostomies have traditionally been placed at the time of surgical exploration and should still be placed that way if there is a significant possibility of future malignant bowel obstruction. The additional operative morbidity is very low and, if needed, the benefits are considerable. Current available technology now makes laparotomy for the sole purpose of placement of a gastrostomy unnecessary, but its liberal use during laparotomy should still be advocated. Patients with malignant bowel obstruction which is not amenable to surgical correction should be considered for venting percutaneous gastrostomy (48, 49). New methods and technologies make placement very safe and even patients with extensive intraperitoneal disease, previous surgery, or ascites can be considered (50). There are currently no absolute contra-indications to percutaneous gastrostomy, if the clinical situation mandates it.

The history of percutaneous gastrostomy dates back to the early 1980s when two separate technologies emerged, both based on the expanding availability of fiber optic endoscopy and advances in interventional radiology. Gauderer et al. developed a technique whereby the stomach was insufflated and then cannulated percutaneously and a string passed to a waiting gastroscope in the stomach (51). This string was then pulled out the esophagus and used to advance a gastrostomy tube, external position first, back through the mouth, esophagus, and stomach, and out the previous skin opening. The gastric portion of the tube contains a fixed T-bar which prevents accidental dislodgment of the tube, but also necessitates repeat gastroscopy and removal or change of tubes. These tubes are especially well suited for patients who are less than fully cooperative with their care. It provides excellent decompression of the upper GI tract and can be used for nutrition as well.

An alternative technique was described by Russell *et al.* (52) and is based on the methods of Seldinger. As with the Gauderer technique, the stomach is insufflated with a gastroscope and a percutaneous needle used to cannulate the stomach. Next, a guide wire is advanced into the stomach, its presence verified by the endoscopist, and the needle exchanged from an introducer with a peel-away sheath. The wire and introducer are removed, a balloon tip tube advanced through the introducer, and the introducer peeled away. The balloon is inflated, seated against the abdominal wall, and the position once again verified endoscopically. Once a track is established, these tubes are easily exchanged without the need for guide wires, radiology, or endoscopy, but they are more prone to accidental dislodgment. Russell *et al.* (52) reported a 10% minor complication rate in their initial communication and no major complications. Werth *et al.* (53) confirmed these excellent results and reported tube usage for a median of months. The results and complication rates are acceptable with both techniques. The most serious complications are related to intra-abdominal leaks from the stomach and infections at the skin site. It is interesting to note that the majority of patients after uneventful percutaneous gastrostomy placement will demonstrate pneumoperitoneum on computed tomography (CT), with no clinical sequelae (54). Hennigan and Forbes (55) also reported a case of colonic obstruction from a gastrostomy tube. The determination as to which is used should be based on physician experience, patient condition, and available resources.

About the same time that endoscopic techniques were being developed to place a percutaneous gastrostomy tube, interventional radiologists were bringing their evolving skills to bear (56, 57). They were able to show that their complication rates were significantly better than those for surgically placed gastrostomy, and comparable to endoscopic percutaneous methods (58). More recent enhancements of these basic techniques have improved the radiologists' ability to avoid injury to intervening structures. CT guidance allows placement of gastrostomy tubes in patients with previous upper abdominal surgery or obstructing esophageal lesions since the stomach or any overlying interfering structures are exactly localized, often without gastric insufflation or with only esophageal insufflation (59). There is even a report of percutaneous placement of a tube through the left lobe of the liver (60).

Ultrasound guidance of gastrostomy tube placement has recently been reported. Ultrasound is used to map the outline of the left lobe of the liver, and then the insufflated stomach is cannulated percutaneously under fluoroscopy. Interposition of other upper abdominal structures can also be detected. In those patients who are not completely obstructed or those with esophageal obstruction, venting gastrostomies can be used for nutrition or hydration. Some patients with gastro esophageal reflux (GER) may benefit from conversion of their percutaneous gastrostomies to percutaneous gastrojejunostomies, decreasing the risk of GER and allowing the safe reinstitution of enteral hydration or nutrition (61–63).

Jejunostomy

Table 10.6 shows indications for percutaneous endoscopic gastrostomy (PEG) and percutaneous endoscopic jejunostomy (PEJ) placement. Patients with significant GER are at risk for aspiration pneumonia when gastric feeding is used. In such patients, jejunal feedings are considered ideal. The infusion rate into a PEJ usually should not exceed 150ml/h as the jejunum lumen does not have the same reservoir capacity as the stomach.

Table 10.6 Indications for PEG and PEJ tube placement

Primary neurologic disorders
Oropharyngeal disorders
Esophageal/gastric obstruction
Nutritional supplementation (anorexia)
Gastroparesis
Recurrent aspiration
Benign esophageal disorders
Malignant tracheoesophageal fistula

Jejunal feedings are usually implemented by operative jejunostomy or by means of a long nasojejunal tube. Ponsky and Aszodi (64) set up a new method for the establishment of a feeding jejunostomy in combination with a decompressing gastrostomy. In this way it is possible to maintain nutrition with concomitant prevention of GER.

Numerous operative techniques for the establishment of enteral access have been developed. Such techniques are quite successful but are associated with a complication incidence ranging from 3 to 35% (65).

Bozzetti *et al.* described a new method to provide EN via a tube inserted into the jejunum and then connected to a Port-a-Cath lodged in a subcutaneous pocket without any external device (66). The authors sum up the advantages of their technique as follows.

1. If an external feeding ostomy is decided upon during an operation, a subcutaneous jejunostomy (SJ) can be performed easily with less discomfort to the patient and it does not alter their self-image.

2. SJ can be placed as a prophylactic procedure in patients at risk of developing intractable gastric or proximal small-bowel obstruction in the course of their disease.

3. SJ can be managed in two ways. If the patient would like to avoid alterations of his or her body image, liquid feeding can be carried out by using the Port-a-Cath and a Huber needle size 19 G together with an infusion pump. In this case patients and/or relatives have to be properly trained for the safe and sterile maintenance of the system. Alternatively, with a simple skin incision under local anesthesia, the Port-a-Cath can be exteriorized and disconnected from the tube and the tube can be used as the usual catheter jejunostomy.

Percutaneous endoscopic jejunostomy can be performed as a modification of PEG involving transpyloric passage of a small bore feeding tube under endoscopic guidance to provide alimentation directly into the small bowel (67–72). Table 10.7 shows indications for PEJ with respect to PEG.

Table 10.7 Indications for PEJ versus PEG

Aspirations in patients with PEG
Chronic intermittent vomiting
Delayed gastric emptying
Gastroesophageal reflux
Previous partial or total gastrectomy
Neuromuscular dysfunction resulting from
   injury to the spinal cord or head

The technique is simple and is carried out percutaneously in the endoscopy suite using a topical anesthetic (1% lidocaine) and intravenous diazepam (5–10 mg) or midazolam (2–4 mg). Placement of the PEG tube, followed by the introduction of the PEJ tube, requires approximately 20–30 minutes.

Ponsky *et al.* (73) reported that in their series of 307 percutaneous gastrostomies and 16 percutaneous jejunostomies performed on 80 children and 242 adults, a 0.3% mortality and 5.9% morbidity resulted, but no long-term follow-up was reported.

The data in literature concerning long-term follow-up are not encouraging. Kaplan *et al.* (74) reported their experience on the placement and long-term follow-up of 26 PEJ tubes (Microvasive PEJ tube) in 23 patients (21 with neurologic disorders and two with cancer) over a 2-year period. In three patients a second PEJ tube was inserted after the first one failed. There was no mortality related to the placement of the PEJ tube. The number of episodes of aspiration pneumonia during an equal time interval were 13 with nasogastric tube (in six patients), 11 episodes with PEG, after conversion of PEJ to PEG tube feeding (in seven patients) and five with PEJ (in four patients). Two patients died from aspiration pneumonia less than 1 week after the PEJ tube had failed and had been converted to a PEG tube. Of the 26 PEJ tubes, 22 (84%) failed and had been functional for an average of only 39.5 days (range 1–480 days). The reasons for failure were separation of the inner PEJ tube from the outer gastrostomy tube (59%), clogging due to the small PEJ tube diameter and the use of crushed tables (32%), and kinking and knotting (9%).

The results of the study showed that there was a high incidence of upper gastrointestinal bleeding (30%) which stopped spontaneously; only one patient needed a transfusion. The etiology of the bleeding was not determined. Forty-eight per cent of the patients in the study died on average 82 days after tube placement.

According to the authors, the high failure rate can be attributed to flaws in the design of the PEJ tubes and the small diameter (the internal diameter was only 3 mm). A two-port tube (Ross/Microvasive) may allow for simultaneous gastric administration of medications and PEJ tube feeding and avoid the detachment of the PEJ tube. However, as the diameter of both ports is still very small, clogging still remains a problem.

The results of the study by DiSario *et al.* (75) of 20 malnourished patients where PEG was converted to a PEJ for various reasons are also not encouraging. The PEG tube placement followed by the introduction of the PEJ tube, required 60 minutes on average.

Serious complications occurred in 95% of the patients: aspiration (17 episodes in 12 patients of whom eight died), regurgitation/reflux (15 episodes in seven patients), and gastrointestinal bleeding (four episodes in three patients) thus necessitating transfusions. Seven patients had more than one complication. Sixty-seven per cent of the patients where PEJ had been placed with the sole aim of preventing aspiration continued to aspirate after the catheter was placed. The catheter tip may have been placed in the duodenum in some patients with successive passage into the stomach which had then brought about aspiration.

The PEJ tube failed in 14 patients (70%) due to occlusion (27 episodes in nine patients), malposition (nine episodes in seven patients), leakage at the PEG–PEJ junction (nine episodes in six patients), extrusion (six episodes in three patients), cracking (two episodes in two patients), kinking (two episodes in two patients), or rupture of the catheter (two episodes in two patients). Because of these complications the tube did not function for 18% of the time. The 30 day mortality rate attributable to PEG–PEJ was 25%. Interestingly the study suggests that enteral feeding through a PEJ does not prevent aspiration even though this technique had always been indicated for patients at risk for aspiration.

Shailesh *et al.* (76) came to the same conclusion because in their series of six patients with neurological disorders aspiration continued notwithstanding the PEJ, causing the death of three patients. In this report the intra-operative mortality rate was 15.2% and the overall complication rate was 25% (14% non-aspiration related). Wolfsen *et al.* (77) reported a 5% incidence of aspiration with PEG compared with 17% with PEJ. Tube dysfunction occurred in 53% of patients in the PEJ group compared with 24% in the PEG group. Thus, PEJ not only failed to prevent aspiration but it is also associated with a higher incidence of aspiration and tube failure or dysfunction.

This shows that, in clinical practice, follow-up studies are always necessary in order to evaluate the efficacy, tolerability, and complications deriving from any therapy or new technique. According to Lewis (78) the only way to ensure that reflux or aspiration from tube feeding does not occur is to place the tip of the tube beyond the ligament of Treitz.

It may be possible that the incidence of aspiration could be lower after surgical jejunostomy compared with percutaneous endoscopic jejunostomy, but at present there is no available comparable data.

According to Adams *et al.* (79) jejunostomy is not an innocuous procedure; it carries a substanial risk of complications and death. Feeding jejunostomy should be performed only in patients with clear indications and where there is a high potential for long-term use or in those where gastrostomy is not feasible.

Colostomy

Malignant obstruction of the colon not amenable to definitive surgical correction is generally managed with colonic diversion just proximal to the obstructing lesion.

Thus, the best palliation for obstruction from a rectal carcinoma or invasive gynecological malignancy is an end-sigmoid colostomy. Left-sided lesion will occasionally be easily handled by a loop-transverse colostomy, but lesions more proximal than the mid-transverse colon are best handled with an end-ileostomy rather than a right-sided colostomy. These are difficult to construct and difficult to care for. Placement of the stoma should anticipate further progression of the disease, or further palliative therapy which might affect the bowel involved, such as pelvic irradiation for pain. In such an instance the stoma may be placed higher or more proximal to avoid encroachment by either disease or side-effects of therapy. Generally, two basic principles of stoma construction apply. First, make the most distal stoma possible, since dehydration will be less and stoma care easier. Second, while complete distal obstruction might make a double-barrel or loop stoma necessary, end-stomas are usually much easier to care for and provide a higher quality of life.

The site of decompression in complete colonic obstruction is often dictated not by the site obstruction but rather colonic geometry. Since the luminal diameter of the cecum is the largest in the colon, La Place's law dictates the greatest wall tension in this structure, and it is often the most vulnerable to distending forces. The desire to protect the vulnerable cecum and provide the most efficient diversion of ileal effluent has led to some enthusiasm for cecal decompression, either cecostomy or tube cecostomy. Cecal-cutaneous anastomosis, or blow hole cecostomy, requires a mini-laparotomy, and is a very difficult stoma to care for and, while it may still have a role in high-risk patients prior to definitive surgery, it has little role as definitive decompression (80). Tube cecostomy can be done operatively or percutaneously and has had good results in small series (81), but overall is still fraught with technical difficulties and complications (82–84).

Those patients with malignant, irreversible colonic obstruction are best managed medically or with an end-ileostomy, which is much easier to construct and care for. Finally, it is important to realize that the quality of life for patients with stomas of all types has been immeasurably improved by the efforts of enterostomal therapy nurses. They are well trained and experienced in the care of all stomas, good and bad, and can be of great value to patients with stomas of less than optimal construction because of their disease. They should be an essential component of any unit that cares for large numbers of patients with malignant bowel obstruction.

Rectal intubation

Anatomically, the penultimate method of decompression of the gastrointestinal tract is a rectal tube, and rectal intubation serves an important role in the treatment of colonic pseudo-obstruction. Its role in the treatment of obstructing low rectal or anal canal malignant lesions is much less important, whereas proximal diversion or transanal fulguration provide much better palliation.

Conclusions

Evidence from controlled clinical trials suggests that the main benefits of artificial nutrition are the maintenance of or prevention of further deterioration in the nutritional state rather than the restoration of a normal nutritional status. Before starting EN in a cachectic patient we should ask ourselves if and how much this syndrome is the cause of the patient's suffering and what can improve in the patient's life if the progressive worsening is avoided. Would they live longer? Would they live better?

As many patients die due to causes other than cachexia and malnutrition, nutritional support will have a limited role in time. This has to be weighed up with the discomfort and complications that artificial nutrition via gastroenteral intubation, PEG, and PEJ can produce.

The routine use of artificial nutrition should be discouraged. These techniques may be useful in certain cases such as in advanced cancer patients who present hunger symptoms but cannot feed themselves, in patients who will die due to malnutrition before the spreading of cancer, and in those whose sufferance is mainly caused by nutritional deterioration. These techniques may also have a psychological role in patients who want to be fed because they consider food a means of survival. The advantages and disadvantages should be discussed with the patient and his/her family members. Studies evaluating the quality of life among the different techniques of nutritional support systems should be set up.

Any decision regarding the start up or the suspension of artificial feeding in advanced cancer patients should be carried out on a personalized base according to the physical and psychological condition of the single patient, his/her wishes, his/her informed consent, and the patient's clinical situation bearing in mind the prognostic factors of survival. Artificial feeding should not be used indiscriminately as it may lead to serious complications and may even prolong the suffering in some patients with severe or terminal illness.

While tremendous advances have been made in the pharmacologic management of malignant bowel obstruction, decompression of the GI tract can dramatically improve a patient's quality of life. Careful patient selection will minimize treatment-related complications and improve results.

REFERENCES

1. Nixon D, Mohih S, Lawson D *et al.* Total parenteral nutrition as an adjunct to chemotherapy of metastatic colorectal cancer. Cancer Treat Rep 1981;65:121–3.
2. Theologides A. Cancer cachexia. Cancer 1979;43:2004–20.
3. Bruera E, MacDonald RN. Nutrition in cancer patients: an update and review of our experience. J Pain Symptom Manage 1988;3:134–40.
4. Ambrus JL, Ambrus CM, Mink IB. Causes of death in cancer patients. J Med 1975;6:61–4.
5. Inagaki J, Rodriguez V, Bodey GP. Causes of death in cancer patients. Cancer 1974;33:568–73.
6. Klastersky J, Daneau D, Verhest A. Causes of death in patients with cancer. Eur J Cancer 1972;8:149–54.
7. DeWys WD, Begg C, Lavin PT *et al.* Prognostic effect of weight loss prior to chemotherapy in cancer patients. Am J Med 1980;69:491–7.
8. Belghiti J, Longonnet F, Bourstyn E *et al.* Surgical implications of malnutrition and immunodeficiency in patients with carcinoma of the oesophagus. Br J Surgery 1983;70:339–41.
9. Bozzetti F, Migliavacca S, Scotti A *et al.* Impact of cancer, type, site, stage and treatment on the nutritional status of patients. Ann Surgery 1982;196:170–9.

10. Fein R, Kelsen DP, Geller N. *et al.* Adenocarcinoma of the esophagus and gastroesophageal function: prognostic factors and results of therapy. Cancer 1985;56:2512–18.
11. Bruera E. Current pharmacological management of anorexia in cancer patients. Oncology 1992;6(1):125–9.
12. Brennan M. Nutritional support. In: Cancer, principles and practice of oncology (ed. De Vita VT, Hellman S, Rosenberg SA). Philadelphia: Lippincott, 1985;1907–20.
13. Theologides A. Anorexins, asthenins and cachectins in cancer. Am J Med 1986;81: 296–8.
14. Bodnar R, Pasternak G, Mann P *et al.* Mediation of anorexia by human recombinant tumor necrosis factor through a peripheral action in the rat. Cancer Res 1989;49:6280–4.
15. Masuno H, Yoshimura H, Ogana N *et al.* Isolation of lyolytic factor (toxohormon-L) from ascites fluid of patients with hepatoma and its effect on feeding behaviour. Eur J Cancer Clin Oncol 1984;20:1177–85.
16. Kris M, Gralla R. Management of vomiting caused by anticancer drugs. Adv Pain Res Ther 1990;16:337–44.
17. Manara L, Bianchetti A. The central and peripheral influence of opioids on gastrointestinal propulsion. Ann Rev Pharmacol Toxicol 1985;75:249–73.
18. Alexander HR, Norton JA. Pathophysiology of cancer cachexia. In: Oxford textbook of palliative medicine (ed. Doyle, D, Hanks, GWC, MacDonald, N). Oxford University Press Inc, New York 1993;316–29.
19. Brescia F, Adler D, Gray G, Ryan M, Cimino J, Mamtani R. Hospitalized advanced cancer patients. J Palliat Care 1991;7:25–9.
20. Bruera E, Fainsinger RL. Clinical management of cachexia and anorexia. In: Oxford textbook of palliative medicine (ed. Doyle, D, Hanks, GWC, MacDonald, N). Oxford University Press Inc, New York 1993;330–7.
21. Bernstein I. Etiology of anorexia in cancer. Cancer 1986;58:1881–6.
22. Bozzetti F. Effects of artificial nutrition on the nutritional status of cancer patients. J Parent Ent Nutr 1989;13:406–20.
23. Ginsberg GG, Lipman TO. Nutritional support and therapy in GI disease: an overview. Prac Gastroenterol 1992;16(5):20–32.
24. Randall H. Enteral nutrition: tube feeding in acute and chronic illness. J Parent Ent Nutr 1984;8:113–34.
25. Burt M, Gorschboth C, Brennan M. A controlled prospective, randomized trial evaluating the metabolic effects of enteral and parenteral nutrition in the cancer patient. Cancer 1982;49:1092–105.
26. McArdle AH, Palmason C, Morency I, Brown RA. A rationale for enteral feeding as the preferable route for hyperalimentation. Surgery 1981;90/4:616–23.
27. Maltoni M, Pirovano M, Lanni O, Labianca R, Amadori D. Prognostic factors in terminal cancer patients. Eur J Palliat Care 1994;1/3:122–5.
28. Maltoni M, Nanni O, Derni S *et al.* Clinical prediction of survival is more accurate than the Karnofsky performance status in estimating life span of terminally ill cancer patients. Eur J Cancer 1994;30(6):764–6.
29. Bozzetti F (chairperson), Amadozi D, Bruera E *et al.* Guidelines on artificial nutrition versus hydration in terminal cancer patients. Report of an *ad hoc* consensus conference. Nutrition, in press. 1996.
30. Fainsinger RL, MacEachern T, Miller MJ *et al.* The use of hypodermoclysis for rehydration in terminally ill cancer patients. J Pain Symptom Manage 1994;9:298–302.
31. Nelson JK, Palumbo PJ, O'Brien PC. Home enteral nutrition: observations of a newly established programme. Nutr Clin Pract 1986;1:193–6.
32. Bozzetti F. Is enteral nutrition a primary therapy in cancer patients? Gut 1994;(Suppl 1):35:S65–8.
33. Silk DBA, Elia M. Home enteral nutrition: general aspects and a comparison between the United States and Britain. Nutrition 1994;10/2:115–23.

34. Cutie AJ, Altman E, Lenkel L. Compatibility of enteral products with commonly employed drug additives. J Parent Ent Nutr 1983;7:186–7.
35. Bauer LA. Interference of oral phenytoin absorption by continuous nasogastric feedings. Neurology 1982;32:570–2.
36. Saklad J, Graves RH, Sharp WP. Interaction of oral phenytoin with enteral feedings. J Parent Ent Nutr 1986;10:322–4.
37. Pichard C. Choix et usage optimal du materiel pour l'alimentation enterale. In: Des annees a savourer. Nutrition et qualite' de vie de la personne agee. (sour la direction de Charles-Henri Rapin). Editions Payot Lausanne, France 1993;164–7.
38. Payne-James JJ, Rees RGP, Silk DBA. 7g weighted versus unweighted polyurethane nasoenteral tubes—spontaneous transpyloric passage and clinical performance: a controlled trial. Clin Nutr 1990;9:109–12.
39. Silk DBA, Rees RG, Keohane PP. Clinical efficiency and design changes of "fine bore" nasogastric feeding tubes: a seven-year experience involving 809 intubations in 403 patients. J Parent Ent Nutr 1987;11:383–7.
40. Rees RGP, Payne-James JJ, King C, Silk DBA. Spontaneous transpylorus passage and performance of fine bore polyurethane feeding under a controlled clinical trial. J Parent Ent Nutr 1988;12:469–72.
41. Ciocon JO, Silverstone FA, Graver M, Foley CJ. Tube feeding in elderly patients. Arch Int Med 1988;148:429–33.
42. Savassi-Rocha PR, Conceica SA, Ferreira JT *et al.* Evaluation of the routine use of the nasogastric tube in digestive operation by a prospective controlled study. Surgery, Gynecol Obstet 1992;174:317–20.
43. Baines M. The pathophysiology and management of malignant intestinal obstruction. In: Oxford textbook of palliative medicine (ed. Doyle, D, Hanks, GWC, MacDonald, N), Oxford University Press Inc, New York 1993;311–16.
44. Pictus D, Marx MV, Weyman PJ. Chronic intestinal obstruction: value of percutaneous gastrostomy tube placement. Am J Radiol 1988;150:295–7.
45. Ripamonti C. Management of bowel obstruction in advanced cancer. Curr Opin Oncol 1994;6:351–7.
46. Luetzow AM, Chaffoo RA, Young H. Percutaneous gastrostomy: the Stanford experience. Laryngoscope 1988;98(10):1035–9.
47. Stellato TA, Gauderer MW. Percutaneous endoscopic gastrostomy for gastrointestinal decompression. Ann Surgery 1987;205(2):119–22.
48. van Ooijen B, van der Burg ME, Plantin AS, Siersema PD, Wiggers T. Surgical treatment or gastric drainage only for intestinal obstruction in patients with carcinoma of the ovary or peritoneal carcinomatosis of other origin. Surgery, Gynecol Obstet 1993;176(5):469–74.
49. Gemlo B, Rayner AA, Lewis B *et al.* Home support of patients with end-stage malignant bowel obstruction using hydration and venting gastrostomy. Am J Surgery 1986;152:100–4.
50. Lee MJ, Saini S, Brink JA, Morrison MC, Hahn PF, Mueller PR. Malignant small bowel obstruction and ascites: not a contraindication to percutaneous gastrostomy. Clin Radiol 1991;44(5):332–4.
51. Gauderer MW, Ponsky JL, Izant RJ,Jr. Gastrostomy without laparotomy: a percutaneous endoscopic technique. J Pediatr Surgery 1980;15(6):872–5.
52. Russell TR, Brotman M, Norris F. Percutaneous gastrostomy. A new simplified and cost-effective technique. Am J Surgery 1984;148(1):132–7.
53. Werth B, Meyer B, Beglinger C, Stalder G. Percutaneous endoscopic gastrostomy. Personal experiences with Russell's method. (German). J Suisse Med 1989;119(17):527–31.
54. Wojtowycz MM, Arata JA,Jr, Micklos TJ, Miller FJ,Jr. CT findings after uncomplicated percutaneous gastrostomy. Am J Roentgenol 1988;151(2):307–9.
55. Hennigan TW, Forbes A. Colonic obstruction caused by endoscopic percutaneous gastrostomy. Eur J Surgery 1992;158(8):435.
56. Wills JS, Oglesby JT. Percutaneous gastrostomy. Radiology 1983;149(2):449–53.

57. van Sonnenberg E, Wittich GR, Cabrera OA *et al.* Percutaneous gastrostomy and gastroenterostomy: 2. Clinical experience. Am J Roentgenol 1986;146(3):581–6.
58. Ho CS, Yee AC, McPherson R. Complications of surgical and percutaneous nonendoscopic gastrostomy: review of 233 patients (see comments). Gastroenterology 1988;95(5):1206–10.
59. Sanchez RB, van Sonnenberg E, D'Agostino HB, Goodacre BW, Moyers P, Casola G. CT guidance for percutaneous gastrostomy and gastroenterostomy. Radiology 1992;184(1): 201–5.
60. Kanazawa S, Naomoto Y, Mitani M *et al.* Percutaneous transhepatic gastrostomy with CT guidance in patients with partial gastrectomy. (Japanese.) Nippon Acta Radiol 1993;53(12):1380–6
61. Olson DL, Krubsack AJ, Stewart ET. Percutaneous enteral alimentation: gastrostomy versus gastrojejunostomy. Radiology 1993;187(1):105–8).
62. Hicks ME, Surratt RS, Pictus D, Marx MV, Lang EV. Fluoroscopically guided percutaneous gastrostomy and gastroenterostomy: analysis of 158 consecutive cases. Am J Roentgenol. 1990;154(4):725–8.
63. Ho CS, Yeung EY. Percutaneous gastronomy and transgastric jejunostomy. (Review.) Am J Roentgenol 1992;158(2):251–7.
64. Ponsky JL, Aszodi A. Percutaneous endoscopic jejunostomy. Am J Gastroenterol 1984;79/ 2:113–16.
65. Torosian MH, Rombeau JL. Feeding by tube enterostomy. Surgery Gynecol Obstet 1980;150:918–27.
66. Bozzetti F, Bignami P, Cozzaglio L. Subcutaneous jejunostomy. J Parent Ent Nutr 1992;16/ 3:286–8.
67. Alberti-Flor JJ, Dunn GD. A modified feeding jejunostomy tube to use with the percutaneous endoscopic technique. Am J Gastroenterol 1985;80:400.
68. Gotfreid EB, Plumser AB. Endoscopic gastrojejunostomy technique to establish small bowel feeding without laparotomy. Gastrointest Endoscop 1984;30:355–7.
69. Lewis B, Mauer K, Bush A. The rapid placement of jejunal feeding tubes: the Seldinger technique applied to the gut. Gastrointest Endoscop 1990;36:730–40.
70. Wadiwala IM, Bacon BR. A simplified technique for constructing a feeding jejunostomy from an existing gastrostomy. Gastrointest Endoscop 1986;32:288–90.
71. Shike M, Schroy P, Ritchie MA, Lightdale CJ, Morse R. Percutaneous endoscopic jejunostomy in cancer patients with previous gastric resection. Gastrointest Endoscop 1987;33:372–4.
72. Shike M, Wallach C, Bloch A, Brennan MF. Combined gastric drainage and jejunal feeding through a percutaneous endoscopic stoma. Gastrointest Endoscop 1990;36(3):290–2.
73. Ponsky JL, Gauderer MWL, Stellato TA, Aszodi A. Percutaneous approaches to enteral alimentation. Am J Surgery 1985;149:102–5/
74. Kaplan DS, Murthy UK, Linscheer WG. Percutaneous endoscopic jejunostomy: long-term follow-up of 23 patients. Gastrointest Endoscop 1989;35/5:403–6.
75. DiSario JA, Foutch PG Sankowski RA. Poor results with percutaneous endoscopic jejunostomy. Gastrointest Endoscop 1990;36:257–60.
76. Shailesh LTC, Kadakia C, Sullivan HO, Starnes E. Percutaneous endoscopic gastrostomy or jejunostomy and the incidence of aspiration in 79 patients. Am J Surgery 1992;164:114–18.
77. Wolfsen HC, Kozarek RA, Ball TJ, Patterson DJ, Botoman VA. Tube dysfunction following percutaneous endoscopic gastrostomy and jejunostomy. Gastrointest Endoscop 1990;36:261–3.
78. Lewis B, Perform PEJ, not PED. Editorial. Gastrointest Endoscop 1990;36:311–13.
79. Adams MB, Seabrook GR, Quebbeman EA, Condon RE. Jejunostomy. A rarely indicated procedure. Arch Surgery 1986;121:236–8.
80. Gurke L, Marx A, Rothenbuhler JM, Harder F. Is cecostomy still current for emergency relief of the colon? (German.) Helvet Chirurgica Acta 1991;57(6):961–4.

81. Morrison MC, Lee MJ, Stafford SA, Saini S, Mueller PR. Percutaneous cecostomy: controlled transperitoneal approach. Radiology 1990;176(2):574–6.
82. Kristiansen VB, Sorensen C, Kjaergaard J, Jensen HE. Cecostomy can not be recommended as a routine method in the treatment of acute left-sided obstructive colon cancer. (Danish.) Ugeskrift for Laeger 1990;152(2):101–3.
83. Rosenberg L, Gordon PH. Tube cecostomy revisited. Can J Surgery 1986;29(1):38–40.
84. Maginot TJ, Cascade PN. Abdominal wall cellulitis and sepsis secondary to percutaneous cecostomy. Cardiovasc Interven Radiol 1993;16(5):328–31.

11

Cachexia in context: the interactions among anorexia, pain, and other symptoms

Jane Ingham and Russell Portenoy

INTRODUCTION

Most patients with advanced cancer experience multiple physical and psychological symptoms. Surveys of these patients have begun to clarify symptom prevalence and characteristics, but the methodologies used have not greatly illuminated the many potential interactions among them. Although it is apparent that symptom interactions are common, the types of relationships that occur in association with any specific symptom, such as anorexia, have not been systematically investigated. Given that these interactions probably have both diagnostic and therapeutic implications, the effort to elucidate the most salient is clearly justified. The following discussion first reviews symptom prevalence and the evidence for the existence of various types of symptom interactions in this group of patients. Pain and anorexia are emphasized to illustrate these potential interactions. Methodological issues that are relevant in the assessment of these symptom interactions are then discussed. This analysis provides a foundation for an approach to symptom assessment that recognizes the potential therapeutic implications of these interactions.

SYMPTOM PREVALENCE AND INTERACTIONS

Numerous surveys have documented the high prevalence of symptoms in patients with advanced cancer (1–10). Many symptoms have prevalence rates greater than 50% (Table 1.1). Most patients experience multiple symptoms, a phenomenon that has been directly confirmed in several surveys (3, 4, 10).

Fatigue (or weakness), pain, and anorexia are the most prevalent symptoms across surveys (2–10). Direct comparison of one survey to another is difficult, however, due to the diversity of symptoms reported, differing methods of data collection, and problems relating to the taxonomy of symptomatology. The finding that the most common symptoms are generally considered to be 'physical' (for example, pain, fatigue, or nausea) can be ascribed to a methodology that often does not address psychological symptomatology. Depressed mood and anxiety have been found to be extremely common when specific inquiries have been made (10) and surveys that have applied specific psychological measures have repeatedly observed high prevalence rates for psychological symptoms (11–13).

Table 11.1 Prevalence of symptoms in advanced cancer

Symptoms	Reuben et al. (9) (n=1592) Patient or primary carer interview[a] %	Grosvenor et al. (6) (n=254) Patient interview[b] %	Dunlop et al. (5) (n=50) Patient interview[c] %	Ventafridda et al. (7) (n=115) Patient question-naire[a] %	Fainsinger et al. (8) (n=100) Review of patient or nurse rated symptoms record[c] %	Curtis et al. (3) (n=100) Patient question-naire[a] %	Portenoy et al. (10) (n=243) Prospective patient rated data[b] %
Lack of energy						32	74
Fatigue						40	
Pain	51	27 [abd]	46	59	99	89	64
Weakness			82	51		36	
Sleepiness			4	13		7	60
Insomnia			46	16		28	52
Confusion	12		30	6	39		
Nervous feeling				39			61
Depression		52				31	
Dyspnea	53		30	10	46	41	24
Cough			28	6			28
Anorexia	79		58	30		55	44
Nausea	44	39	42	6	71	32	44
Taste change		46				26	35
Dry mouth	73	41	68	30		40	54
Vomiting		27	32	4		25	21
Constipation	54	41	36	23		40	35
Weight loss	75					58	27
Edema			46			11	27
Sweating	28			14			40
Worrying							71
Feeling sad				57			65

N.B. Surveys involving patient interviews. Symptoms are recorded if any two surveys demonstrated a prevalence of greater than 25% or if any one survey demonstrated a prevalence of 50% or more for an individual symptom.

All surveys were specifically undertaken in patients with advanced cancer with the exception of Portenoy et al. where although two-thirds had metastatic cancer, patients with early disease were also included.

[a] Hospice or palliative care in patients and home care patients.
[b] Cancer center in- and out-patients.
[c] Hospice or palliative care in-patients only.

The challenge inherent in the clinical assessment of symptoms and their interactions is evident in the complex findings related to the most prevalent symptoms. For example, although most surveys report that fatigue is the most common symptom in the population with advanced cancer, occurring with a prevalence of 40–70% (1, 3–5, 7, 10, 11), the complaint of fatigue may actually reflect the presence of several other related symptoms. Patients use 'fatigue' to describe lack of energy or vitality, muscle weakness, tiredness, or sleepiness. The underlying pathology can be as different as severe anemia and major depression. It is apparent, therefore, that fatigue is multidimensional and further studies of patients with this complaint are needed to clarify the nature of this problem. In the clinical setting, a report of fatigue requires careful assessment to ascertain the type of problem and its causes.

Table 11.2   Mean prevalence of pain in common advanced cancers[a]

Type of cancer	Mean prevalence
Lung	72
Colon	69
Breast	72
Prostate	70
Urinary tract	65
Uterus/cervix	72
Lymphoma	58
Oral/pharynx	66
Pancreas	79
Leukemia	52

[a] Modified from Bonica, (15). The mean prevalence was obtained by computing data from three to six reports, containing data on each specific tumor.

Pain is experienced by approximately one-third of all cancer patients and by approximately 70–90% of those with advanced cancer (14–16). The prevalence of pain varies with the specific tumor type (15) (Table 11.2). It is most prevalent in tumors that commonly involve bone or neural plexi and is least prevalent in the hematological malignancies. The latter finding is consistent with the observation that cancer pain is usually associated with a site of ongoing damage to somatic or visceral tissues or with a clearly defined neuropathic mechanism. None the less, it is also evident that pain perception is strongly influenced by psychological factors related to mood and cognition (17). In one large survey, significant pain was experienced by 39% of cancer patients who had a specific psychiatric diagnosis and only 19% of those without a psychiatric diagnosis (18). The report of pain cannot be adequately assessed without consideration of its relationship to other symptomatology.

A recent survey of pain in ambulatory patients with lung or colon cancer illustrated the complexity of symptoms and their relationships to both other symptoms and quality of life (19). Prospective interviews revealed that 'persistent or frequent' pain was experienced by 33% of patients. Pain interfered moderately or more with general activity and work in approximately half of the patients; more than half reported moderate or greater pain interference with sleep, mood, and enjoyment of life. Mood contributed independently and significantly to the variance in average pain intensity and more than half of the variance in a derived measure of pain interference with function was explained by the mood score and some of the pain descriptors (for example, frequency, intensity, and number of pains). Thus, the assessment of symptoms can be complicated, incorporating many aspects other than prevalence.

The prevalence of anorexia in advanced cancer is in the range of 30–79% (2, 3, 5, 7, 9–11), (See Chapter 5). Clinical experience suggests that the presence of gastro-intestinal symptomatology is related to anorexia and that anorexia is related to cachexia. Gastrointestinal symptoms that may influence appetite and caloric intake include difficulty with swallowing, xerostomia, taste change, early satiety, dyspepsia, nausea, bloating, and constipation (3, 5–10, 20). Surveys have demonstrated that these symptoms are highly prevalent in the cancer population (Table 11.3). Anorexia may also occur in association with other symptoms, such as depressed mood.

The relationship between specific gastrointestinal symptoms and weight loss in patients with advanced cancer has been addressed in only one study (6), which included patients with a variety of malignancies (68% had primary neoplasms unrelated to the gastrointestinal tract). Although chronic gastrointestinal and oropharyngeal symptomatology occurred in the majority of patients, abdominal fullness, taste changes, mouth dryness, and vomiting occurred more frequently in the group with weight loss. Although the prevalence of anorexia was not specifically addressed in this survey, the data support the clinical impression that symptom complexes related to gastrointestinal function (probably including anorexia) con-tribute to the development of cachexia. These interactions must be considered in both clinical practice and future studies of symptom epidemiology.

Surveys that address the spectrum of psychological symptoms in cancer patients are not common, although a number have documented a high prevalence of psychiatric diagnoses (18, 21, 22). In one survey of 215 hospitalized ambulatory patients at three cancer centers, 47% met the criteria for a psychiatric disorder. Sixty-nine per cent of these patients had an adjustment disorder with anxious or depressed mood and 13% had a major depression; the remainder of those with a psychiatric disorder had organic mental disorder (8%), personality disorder (7%), or anxiety disorder (4%) (18). In many instances psychological symptoms impact on other symptoms, particularly on anorexia and pain.

The prevalence of psychological symptoms overall is undoubtedly higher than the prevalence of specific psychiatric disorders, the diagnosis of which requires that the patient meet published criteria (23). This observation exemplifies the need to recognize lack of 'specificity' as an issue in the assessment of symptom interactions. Many patients present with symptoms that are too transitory or mild to meet criteria for any diagnosis. Others report the presence of only one symptom of a complex that, if experienced together, would fulfil the diagnostic criteria for a particular disorder. For example, a recent survey demonstrated that the prevalence of 'worrying', 'feeling sad', and 'feeling nervous' (71%, 65%, and 61% respectively) far exceeded the prevalence of any psychiatric diagnoses (10). Sadness or anxiety may represent primary psychiatric problems or organic mood disturbances secondary to any of a large number of causes. Psychological symptoms, such as fatigue, pain, anorexia, and other

Table 11.3 Prevalence of gastrointestinal symptoms in advanced cancer

Symptoms	Reuben et al. (9) (n=1592) Patient or primary carer interview[c] %	Grosvenor et al. (6) (n=254) Patient interview[b] %	Dunlop et al. (5) (n=50) Patient interview[c] %	Ventafridda et al. (7) (n=115) Patient questionnaire[a] %	Fainsinger et al. (8) (n=100) Review of patient or nurse rated symptom[c] %	Curtis et al. (3) (n=100) Patient questionnaire[a] %	Portenoy et al. (10) (n=243) Prospective patient rated data[b] %
Nausea	44	39	42	6	71	32	44
Anorexia	79		58	30		55	44
Vomiting		27	32	4		25	21
Dry mouth	73	41	68	30		40	54
Constipation	54	41	36	23		40	35
Swallowing difficulty	43	24		9			11
Diarrhoea	25		4	5			24
Hiccoughs				1			
Early satiety						40	
Taste change		46				26	35
Burping			4				
Dry retching			4				
Salivation			2				
Regurgitation			2				
Indigestion			2				
Weight loss	75						27
Abdominal fullness		61					37
Chewing difficulty		15					
Mouth pain		10					12
Denture problems		16					

N.B. surveys involving patient interviews. Any gastrointestinal symptom that we assessed has been included. Not all symptoms were assessed in each survey.

All surveys were specifically undertaken in patients with advanced cancer with the exception of Portenoy *et el.* where although two-thirds had metastatic cancer, patients with early disease were also included.

[a] Hospice or palliative care in-patients and home care patients.
[b] Cancer center in- and out-patients.
[c] Hospice or palliative care in-patients only.

symptoms, must be viewed in the context of relationships to other symptoms and diverse pathophysiologies. Only when assessed in this context can a diagnosis be made and appropriate treatment initiated. Further research is needed to explore the interactions between psychological symptoms, anorexia, and cachexia.

The complex interaction between symptoms, and between groups of symptoms and the underlying neoplasm, may also increase the difficulty in establishing an accurate diagnosis. For example, the diagnosis of a major depression in physically healthy patients depends heavily on the presence of somatic symptoms, such as anorexia, insomnia, fatigue, weight loss, and psychomotor slowing. As noted, however, anorexia and these other symptoms are extremely common in all groups of cancer patients, including those who are not depressed (Table 11.1). This high prevalence of somatic symptoms reduces their utility as diagnostic criteria for psychatric disorders (12, 13, 24). Although it could be postulated that these symptoms are more severe in cancer patients who have concurrent depression, a study that investigated the relationship between physical and non-physical symptoms of depression in patients with advanced cancer observed no correlation between anorexia or weight loss and the non-physical symptoms of depression (13, 25). Anorexia was associated with physical symptoms, such as insomnia and fatigability, but not with feelings of guilt, worthlessness, or hopelessness. These data suggest an etiology other than depression can generally be found in cancer patients with anorxia and weight loss. From a diagnostic perspective, these somatic complaints must be carefully assessed so that therapeutic intervention can be appropriately directed.

Recent studies have also investigated the relationships between symptoms by addressing their impact on global patient distress and quality of life. The results of these studies provide information relevant to the assessment of symptom interactions. The prevalence of a specific symptom always exceeds the proportion of patients who describe it as highly intense or distressing. More important, perhaps, symptoms that are reported to be 'frequent' or 'severe' may not be reported as highly bothersome or distressing (26). In assessing symptom interactions, the intensity, frequency, and distress associated with each symptom must be addressed to interpret patient's complaints properly. The mere report of a symptom should not be presumed to imply that it is burdensome or in need of treatment.

None the less, a high symptom prevalence is usually associated with a relatively poorer quality of life. For example, a large survey of patients with prostate, colon, breast, or ovarian cancer found that most patients had multiple physical and psychological symptoms (median 11.5, range 0–25) and that the number of symptoms per patient was associated with heightened psychological distress and a poorer quality of life (10). In this study, global symptom distress, which also reflected the presence of multiple symptoms, correlated with both impairment of performance status and a relatively poor quality of life. The presence, therefore, of concurrent symptoms such as pain and anorexia may significantly impair quality of life.

The potential interactions between anorexia–cachexia and other symptoms are outlined in Tables 11.4 and 11.5. These tables provide some examples of the potential impact of these interactions. Although research designed to explore these interactions needs to be undertaken, the evidence available, despite substantial gaps in knowledge, supports the existence of many salient interactions among symptoms. Clinical experience, in addition to the results of many of the surveys of symptom prevalence, justifies an approach to comprehensive patient assessment that incorporates both an awareness and an understanding of symptoms and their complex interactions.

Table 11.4 The potential impact of symptoms on cachexia–anorexia

Effect of symptom	Examples
Symptom may predispose to anorexia–cachexia	
Physical symptoms	Change in taste, dysphagia, pain, nausea
Psychological symptoms	Depression
Symptom may increase the severity of anorexia–cachexia	Nausea, pain, depression

Symptom may increase the burden
    resulting from anorexia–cachexia
	Impairment of quality of life from
	    combination of multiple symptoms

Table 11.5 The potential impact of cachexia–anorexia on other symptoms

Effect of cachexia–anorexia	Examples
Predispose to new symptoms	
Physical	Fatigue
Psychological	Depression
Increase the severity of existing symptoms	Nausea, fatigue, depression

Increase the burden resulting from
    symptoms
	Further impairment of quality of life by
	    compounding symptom effects

CLINICAL GUIDELINES: COMPREHENSIVE ASSESSMENT OF THE ADVANCED CANCER PATIENT

The presence of concurrent symptoms may have significant diagnostic or therapeutic implications. For example, evaluation of the characteristics of individual symptoms and the interactions between groups of symptoms, can elucidate the impact of symptom distress on the quality of life. Such implications must be assessed through a comprehensive patient assessment before a management strategy can be formulated. The assessment process may be conceptualized in several steps, beginning with a review of the available data and culminating in a formulation on which therapy can be based.

Step 1: symptom evaluation and investigation review

The initial step in comprehensive assessement of the patient with advanced cancer involves a complete medical history that reviews the cancer diagnosis, the chronology of significant cancer-related events, and all relevant medical, surgical, and psychiatric problems (Table 11.6). Symptoms may have occurred as a result of therapeutic interventions and this may further influence treatment options. In the course of this assessment, the patient's understanding of his or her current disease status should be assessed.

Table 11.6 Comprehensive assessment – Step 1

Cancer history	Past medical history	Current symptomatology	Psychosocial issues
Diagnosis	Previous illness: medical,	Document each symptom	Family history
Chronology	surgical, and psychiatric	Patient prioritization of	Social resources
Therapeutic	Concurrent medical	symptoms with regard	Impact of disease and
interventions	conditions	to distress, frequency,	symptoms on patient
including	Drug allergies or adverse	and severity	and family
operative	drug reactions.	For each symptom inquire	
procedures,		about:	
chemo- and		chronology,	
radiotherapy		clinical characteristics,	
Patient's knowledge of		degree of distress,	
current extent of disease		impact on function,	
		patient perception of etiology,	
		prior treatment modalities,	
		and their efficacy	
Current medications		System review	
Physical examination			
Assess available laboratory and imaging data			

A thorough assessment of the history and nature of each symptom is an essential element in the evaluation of the patient with multiple symptoms. Each symptom should be documented and assessed in terms of its chronology and clinical characteristics. These characteristics include the frequency and severity of the symptom, its associated degree of distress, and its impact on function. Specific enquiries should attempt to clarify the pathophysiology of symptoms, their impact on function, and the efficacy of prior treatment modalities for each symptom. In this evaluation, function should be defined broadly to include physical performance and psychosocial functioning.

Psychosocial issues must be carefully assessed. As discussed previously, this includes evaluation of the interactions that occur between psychological and 'physical' symptoms. The clinician must also be aware of patients' social resources, including family status, financial situation, and the physical environment in which they live. A knowledge of the patient's and family's previous experience with cancer or other progressive medical disease, may provide useful insights into medical problems, anxiety, and fears.

The patient's understanding of the meaning of symptoms in relation to the disease status may be illuminating. Patients or families may believe that a symptom has greater prognostic implications than it does in reality and experience anxiety as a result. For example, a patient with unstable pain requiring escalating opioid doses may interpret this as indicating that death is imminent. Myoclonus during opioid administration may be misconstrued as a new neurological complication and engender additional anxiety.

Symptom assessment must also include a thorough physical examination and review of the available laboratory and imaging data. Particular attention should be directed towards the system from which the symptom is thought to originate. A limited approach is inadequate, however, since the multiplicity of symptoms cannot be fully assessed without a complete physical examination, including a neurological evaluation. Symptoms such as anorexia, which may be related to gastrointestinal disease, mood disorder, or other factors, particularly require a complete physical and psychological examination. Imaging and laboratory data provide additional evidence for mechanisms that may explain the symptom.

Step 2: assessment of symptom and disease impact

A symptom or its treatment may induce other physical or psychological symptoms, increase the severity of other symptoms, and augment global symptom distress. An adverse impact on overall quality of life may occur through effects on the patient's ability to function or through other less direct processes. For example, pain may induce depression, exacerbate anxiety, aggravate anorexia, interfere with the ability to interact socially, or impair physical performance. These primary and secondary effects must be assessed as they may detract from the overall quality of life (Table 11.7)

Table 11.7 Comprehensive assessment – Steps 2 and 3

Symptom impact	**Disease impact**
Impact of each symptom on:	Impact of:
physical condition	physical limitations
psychological status	prognosis
social interactions	concerns regarding:
Global Symptom Distress — impact of overall	disease or symptom
symptom distress on quality of life	progression
Impact of each symptom on other symptoms	social issues
	financial issues
	existential issues
Diagnostic investigations	**Other assessments**
Symptom specific	Psychosocial
Extent of disease	Functional — Rehabilitative,
	physical, and occupational
	therapy

Anorexia poses a particularly interesting example of the need to focus assessment on the type of interactions that may undermine the quality of life. Anorexia does not itself cause physical discomfort unless accompanied by nausea, yet it is reported as a distressing symptom by one-third to three-quarters of patients (5, 7, 10). Its impact is presumably through secondary physical and psychological effects. It may result in cachexia and malnutrition, which could contribute to fatigue and possibly other problems, such as neuropathy, encephalopathy, and skin problems. The psychological effects include anxiety about the meaning of disinterest in food and its possible consequences. Quality of life may be affected by this heightened anxiety with cultural and family expectations relating to food intake. The cachexia that may attend anorexia can itself be distressing by its effects on self-image. Fear of the consequences of anorexia may also increase the anxiety of the family and other care givers. Therapies used to palliate anorexia, including drugs and physical interventions such as gastrostomy feeding, all have the potential to worsen or alter the patient's symptom profile. These potential interactions suggest that the priority given the management of a symptom like anorexia cannot be considered in terms of the primary effects (weight loss) alone, but also in terms of its secondary physical and psychological effects.

The impact of the underlying disease process must also be considered in this analysis. The disease may directly produce physical impairments, heighten psychological distress, and increase the concern of the family. Anxiety may increase in relation to perceptions as diverse as financial worries and fear of death.

Step 3: diagnostic investigations and specific assessments

To formulate a full understanding of the pathophysiological impact of symptomatology and its relationship to the disease, specific investigations may be required. Radiological or laboratory tests may be appropriate, as may referral for specialist assessment. In a survey that assessed the importance of comprehensive evaluation of patients with cancer pain, it was found that a previously undiagnosed etiology for pain was discovered in 64% of patients who underwent a comprehensive pain assessment (27). Importantly, over 20% of these etiologies were amenable to primary therapy. Specific assessment may also be appropriate to ascertain the requirements for psychosocial support and rehabilitative therapy.

Step 4: assessment of symptom pathophysiology

Clinical inferences about the predominating pathophysiology of a symptom can usually be formulated from the information acquired during the assessment. These inferences, in turn, may clarify important interactions among symptoms (Table 11.8). The complex relationship between pain and anorexia can illustrate the types of interactions that occur and the therapeutic implications of these interactions.

1. Symptoms are concurrent but unrelated in etiology. For example, pain may result from a pathological fracture of the humerus in a patient with metastatic disease to bone and anorexia may be attributed to extensive metastatic disease involving the liver. Treatment of both symptoms should be considered.

2. Symptoms are concurrent and related to the same pathological process. Both abdominal pain and anorexia can occur in a patient with a tumor that results in gastric outlet obstruction. Treatment should be directed where possible at the underlying process as well as at each symptom.

3. Symptoms are concurrent and the second symptom is directly or indirectly a consequence of a pathological process initiated by the other symptom. Chronic pain may initiate depression and associated anorexia. Primary treatment should be intensively focused on the initiating symptom (in this case, pain) and consideration also given to treatment of the other symptom. In the absence of effective treatment directed at the initiating symptom, treatment of the secondary pathological process is likely to be relatively less effective.

4. Symptoms are concurrent and one symptom is a consequence or side-effect of therapy directed against the other. Pain may be treated with opioids, which may cause nausea and anorexia. In this situation, consideration should be given to alternative therapies, dosage, or route modification of the existing therapy, or to treatment of the side-effects of therapy that are resulting in secondary symptoms.

Table 11.8 Comprehensive assessment – Step 4

For each symptom assess:
  inferred pathophysiology
  relationship to other symptoms
    differing pathophysiologies
    same pathophysiology
    casual pathology induced by another symptom
    casual factor is treatment directed at another symptom

The assessment of the patient and the review of investigations provide a framework for a global assessment which addresses the extent of disease and goals of care (Table 11.9). Although the goals of care should, at all stages of disease, encompass symptom

Table 11.9 Comprehensive assessment – Step 5

Global assessment	Prioritize unresolved problems
Clarify:	Clarify the need for:
Extent of disease	further assessment
Goals of care:	primary anti-cancer therapy
Symptom management with or without	symptom palliation — prioritize each
prolongation of life	symptom with respect to patient distress
augmentation of function	functional support
	psychosocial support

management, other priorities may need to be set as well. These relate to therapeutic efforts to improve or retain function, or prolong survival. An informed decision regarding these priorities requires an understanding on the part of the patient or their proxy of the extent of disease and the implications of the symptomatology that is present. Prioritization of major problems should incorporate these goals, which can clarify the need for further assessment and the appropriate level of care.

Step 6: multimodality therapeutic plan

The patient with advanced cancer requires a therapeutic plan that gives consideration to primary anti-cancer therapy, symptom palliation, and therapy directed towards improved physical and psychological function (Table 11.10). A comprehensive symptom assessment allows the clinician to formulate a plan of management that is consistent with the goals of care and integrates symptom management with other treatment imperatives. This plan should be formulated and discussed with the patient.

Table 11.10 Comprehensive assessment – Step 6

Consider each of the following issues.

Primary anti-cancer therapy	Symptom palliation
Type: Chemotherapy Radiation	Direct at most distressing symptoms based on patient prioritization and overall assessment of symptom impact
Surgery Other therapies	Treat etiology where possible, e.g. cancer, concurrent disease, medication, other symptom/s
Impact on disease progression	Employ symptom specific pharmacological therapies
Impact on symptomatology	Monitor and treat side-effects of therapies
	Consider sequential drug trials
	Counsel patient with regard to therapeutic plan, anticipate and advise patient regarding expected outcomes
	Provide regular review and a plan for access to emergency care
Functional approaches	**Psychosocial approaches**
Physical therapies	Psychological/psychiatric therapies
Rehabilitative therapies	Social work assessment, appropriate interventions, and contingency plans
	Pastoral support

Primary anticancer therapy, including chemotherapy, radiation therapy, or surgery, may be appropriate for prevention of disease progression or management or symptomatology even in very advanced disease. Unfortunately, the impact of primary therapies on the quality of life has received limited assessment in clinical trials and there are few data from which to judge the potential benefits and risks of treatments. Although the quality of life assessments at the beginning and end of these therapies may reflect an overall improvement, severe side-effects may occur during therapy (28). Assessment must therefore reflect an understanding of the complexities of symptom interactions if it is to accurately assess quality of life.

Therapies that are symptom directed and not usually considered 'primary' may also be associated with significant burden, including side-effects of medications, financial problems inflicted by the cost of therapies, or difficulties with compliance. Thus, the potential to influence symptomatology in a positive manner must be balanced by the risk that symptom burden will increase. Particularly when life expectancy is short, the hardships associated with treatment may outweigh the benefits. These issues may further increase the complexity of symptom interaction and should not be neglected in treatment decisions.

CONCLUSIONS

In summary, cancer patients frequently experience multiple, concurrent symptoms. The many surveys that provide prevalence rates for the diverse symptoms reported by cancer patients do not yield sufficient information for a comprehensive assessment of the interactions among symptoms in advanced malignancy. Notwithstanding these substantial gaps in knowledge, the evidence available supports the existence of many interactions among symptoms and symptom-directed therapies. Symptoms such as pain and anorexia are extremely prevalent, but the proportion of patients who experience these symptoms as highly distressing, and the complex ways in which the specific characteristics of symptoms may interact with disease-related variables and quality of life are largely unknown. In providing effective care for patients with advanced disease it is essential that a comprehensive assessment address the complex interactions that may occur. The subsequent implementation of appropriate therapeutic interventions depends on this assessment and requires comprehensive ongoing monitoring. Further studies are required to clarify the impact of symptomatology and the interactions among symptoms that occur in this population. The impact of therapies must also be assessed from this perspective. Surveys have been hampered by both the imprecise way in which symptoms are described and the lack of information documenting the dimensions and impact of symptomatology in the individual patient. Further investigations of symptom interactions must be undertaken and should incorporate methodologies designed to assess these factors.

REFERENCES

1. Dunphy KP, and Amesbury BDW. A comparison of hospice and homecare patients: patterns of referral, patient characteristics and predictors on place of death. Palliat Med 1990;4:105–11.
2. Brescia FJ, Adler D, Gray G, Ryan MA, Cimino J, Mamtani R. Hospitalized advanced cancer patients: a profile. J Pain Symptom Manage 1990;5(4):221–7.
3. Curtis EB, Krech R, Walsh TD. Common symptoms in patients with advanced cancer. J Palliat Care 1991;7(2):25–9.
4. Coyle N, Adelhardt J, Foley KM, Portenoy RK. Character of terminal illness in the advanced cancer patient: pain and other symptoms during the last four weeks of life. J Pain Symptom Manage 1990;5(2):83–93.

5. Dunlop GM. A study of the relative frequency and importance of gastrointestinal symptoms and weakness in patients with far advanced cancer. Palliat Med 1989;4:37–43.

6. Grosvenor M, Bulcavage L, Chlebowski RT. Symptoms potentially influencing weight loss in a cancer population. Correlations with primary site, nutritional status, and chemotherapy administration. Cancer 1989;63(2):330–4.

7. Ventafridda V, DeConno F, Ripamonti C, Gamba A, Tamburini M. Quality-of-life assessment during a palliative care programme. Ann Oncol 1990;1(6):415–20.

8. Fainsinger R, Miller MJ, Bruera E, Hanson J, MacEachern T. Symptom control during the last week of life on a palliative care unit. J Palliat Care 1991; 7(1):5–11.

9. Reuben DB, Mor V, Hiriis J. Clinical symptoms and length of survival in patients with terminal cancer. Arch Int Med 1988;148(7):1586–91.

10. Portenoy RK, Thaler HT, Kornblith AB et al. Symptom prevalence, characteristics and distress in a cancer population. Qual Life Res 1994; 3:183–9.

11. McCarthy M. Hospice patients: a pilot study in 12 services. Palliat Med 1990;4:93–104.

12. Plumb M, Holland J. Comparative studies of psychological function in patients with advanced cancer. II. Interviewer-rated current and past psychological symptoms. Psychosom Med 1981;43(3):243–54.

13. Plumb MM, Holland J. Comparative studies of psychological function in patients with advanced cancer — I. Self-reported depressive symptoms. Psychosom Med 1977;39(4):264–76.

14. Portenoy RK. Cancer pain. Epidemiology and syndromes. Cancer 1989; 63(11):2298–307.

15. Bonica JJ. Treatment of cancer pain: current status and future needs. In: Advances in pain research and therapy (ed. Fields HL, Dubner R, and Cervero F). New York: Raven, 1985;589–616.

16. Stjernsward J, Teoh N. The scope of the cancer pain problem. In advances in pain research and therapy, second international congress on cancer pain (ed. Foley KM, Bonica JJ, and Ventafridda V). New York: Raven, 2990;7–12.

17. Portenoy RK. Cancer pain: pathophysiology and syndromes. Lancet, 1992; 339:1026–31.

18. Derogatis LR, Morrow GR, Fetting J et al. The prevalence of psychiatric disorders among cancer patients. JAMA 1983: 249(6): 751–7.

19. Portenoy RK, Miransky J, Thaler HT et al. Pain in ambulatory patients with lung or colon cancer. Prevalence, characteristiics, and effect. Cancer 1992: 70(6):1616–24.

20. Reuben DB, Mor V. Nausea and vomiting in terminal cancer patients. Arch Int med 1986;146(10):2021–3.

21. Levine Pm, Silberfarb PM, Lipowski ZJ. Mental disorders in cancer patients: a study of 100 psychiatric referrals. Cancer 1978;42(3):1385–91

22. Massie MJ, Holland J, Glass E. Delirium in terminally ill cancer patients. Am J Psychiat 1983;140(8):1048–50.

24. Burkberg J, Penman D, Holland JC. Depression in hospitalized cancer patients. Psychosom Med 1984;46(3):199–212.

25. Holland JC, Rowland J, Plumb M. Psychological aspects of anorexia in cancer patients. Cancer Res 1977;;37(7):2425–28.

26. Portenoy RK, Thaler HT, Kornblith AB et al. The Memorial Symptom Assessment Scale: an instrument for the evaluation of symptom prevalence, characteristics, and distress. Eur J Cancer 1994;30(9):1326–36.

27. Gonzales GR, Elliot KJ, Portenoy RK, Foley KM. The impact of a comprehensive evaluation in the management of cancer pain. Pain 1991; 47(2):141)4.

28. Ingham JM, Seidman A, Lepore J et al. The importance of frequent pain measurement in quality of life assessment in cancer clinical trials. Presented at the annual meeting of the American Pain Society, Orlando, Florida. Nov 4, 1993.

12

Psychological impact of cancer cachexia on the patient and family

Irene Higginson and Catherine Winget

PSYCHOLOGICAL DISTRESS IN CANCER

Psychological distress is common among cancer patients and their families. At least 25–50% of cancer patients have sustained psychiatric morbidity in the form of anxiety states, depressive illness, sexual problems, and organic brain syndromes (1). Psychological and psychiatric disorders appear to be more common in patients with advanced cancer and among those who are socially isolated than in the general population (2). Psychological distress and psychiatric disorders have been found in patients shortly after diagnosis (3) and in advanced disease (4–6) with prevalances in the ranges of 10–30 and 10–79% respectively. Psychological distress and psychiatric disorders appear to be common among the family members of patients—indeed, at least two studies have indicated that problems among the spouses are more severe than among patients (2, 7, 8).

Most of these psychological and psychiatric disorders are adjustment disorders or reactive anxiety and depression, but between 6 and 25% of patients have been reported with moderate or severe depression, depending on the stage of disease and the cancer group studied (1–8). Differentiating between an adjustment disorder and a depressive illness can be difficult and may not be necessary, because there is growing evidence that adjustment disorders are successfully managed in a similar way to depression (2). The detection and management of psychological and psychiatric disorders in cancer are described in detail elsewhere (9) and briefly later in this chapter. This chapter reviews the psychological effects and psychological causes of anorexia–cachexia and the psychological components of management.

PSYCHOLOGICAL EFFECTS OF CACHEXIA, ANOREXIA, AND ASTHENIA

In addition to those psychological problems that occur in cancer patients in general, cachexia, anorexia, and asthenia can cause specific additional problems. Anorexia and cachexia have been reported in 40–90% of cancer patients, depending on the definitions used (see Chapters 5 and 11). As treatments to control pain have become more effective and widely used, studies have shown that the symptoms of weakness and fatigue are among the most prevalent towards the end of life occurring in between 50 and 90% of patients (10–12). In some studies, they were described by patients as the most common symptoms causing distress (13).

Variables associated with high distress in a Canadian needs study included poor physical functioning, reduced interest in food and appetite, reduced ability to eat, reduced ability to perform normal activities, fatigue, altered physical appearance, and reduced social relationships (5, 6, 8). It is clear therefore that cachexia, anorexia, and asthenia have a very significant psychological impact.

Anorexia, cachexia, and asthenia can be seen as follows.

1. A sign of impending death (by both the patient and family).

2. A source of conflict between patient and family when a patient becomes unwilling to eat.

3. A barometer of overall condition—because the amount of fluid and food taken is often used to assess this.

Body image

Body image can be affected by many aspects of cancer and its treatment, such as operations and skin reactions to radiotherapy. Cancer cachexia has a considerable impact on a patient's body image. This is the most recognizable external sign of serious illness and is usually a major concern for both patients and families (14, 15). Overall, attractiveness, femininity/masculinity, self-confidence, and having a sense of body integrity may all be important to the concepts of body image, self-image or self-esteem (16).

Studies of students have indicated differences between men and women in their desired body image—over half of the men wanted to be larger, and less than a quarter wanted to be smaller; just the opposite was reported by women (17). While the disturbance in body image may be severe and at times seem out of proportion to any observed disfigurement, this may reflect the measure of distress rather than an irrational appraisal of body image. Furthermore, there is usually no distortion of body size or misperception of body weight among cancer patients, as is found typically in the body image disturbance of anorexia nervosa or bulimia (18).

Altered body image can place a great stress on relationships between partners and it has been suggested that the more accepting a spouse or family member is of the change in appearance the less distress this causes the patient. Conversely, increased anxiety from a family member regarding an altered body image can distress the patient further, in particular if a partner sexually rejects the patient. Patients may avoid dressing and undressing in their partner's presence and have feelings of ugliness, shame or worry about their sexuality. Reactions to changes in body image, for example from surgery, may occur many months later. It has been suggested that there is an initial period of denial about changes in body image, which acts as a defence, so that the reactions can be delayed for a period (18).

Many of the quality of life scales available for cancer patients only assess aspects of body image. Hopwood (18) suggested that the following items are important in the assessment of body image:

(1) dissatisfaction with appearance (distressed);

(2) loss of femininity/masculinity;

(3) reluctance/avoidance to look at self naked;

(4) feeling less attractive or less sexually attractive;

(5) adverse affect of treatment/loss of body integrity;

(6) self-consciousness about appearance;

(7) dissatisfaction with any scar or prosthesis.

Eating as a 'barometer of condition/sign of impending death'

Care givers and patients often connect eating with keeping the person alive (19). In a small descriptive study, Holden (20) found that 12 out of 14 care givers felt that death would result if the patient continued to eat poorly. Comments included: 'Oh, it's very important to eat. He won't be able to live if he doesn't keep his nutrition up, and 'It is so frightening for me to see her lose weight. I knew something was drastically wrong. I blamed myself for not feeding her the right things.'

A patient commented 'If I stop eating, that will be it!'

Nutritional impairment correlates with response to therapy and survival and may be related to the severity of treatment-related toxicity (21, 23). However, a causal relationship has not been proven and it may be that in these studies cachexia–anorexia were symptoms of a more advanced cancer than in those patients without nutritional impairment.

Conflict between patients and their family members

Anorexia has an important emotional significance, because food and eating are essential for survival. Furthermore, the preparation and serving of food is an expression of love and caring. For family members, comfort is often derived from performing this familiar function and when a patient deteriorates and becomes unable to eat, the family member often becomes obsessed with serving something that he/she will eat. If each attempt to eat fails, the family member may feel increasingly rejected, helpless, frustrated and angry (24). Family members may also accuse the patient of giving up and not trying to eat. Food intake can then become a battleground for patients who have been deprived of control in so many other areas of their lives (25). Anxiety over anorexia may be more pronounced in carers than among patients and particularly women carers, because this affects one of their customary roles.

Few studies have examined this in detail and most are only descriptive. Holden (20) studied cancer patients with anorexia and asked patients and family members to describe the patient's actual intake during the two days prior to interview. Twelve out of 14 family members gave information of the amounts of food served compared to what was actually eaten. The prevailing theme of their reports was that the patient was not eating much or not eating well. In contrast, the patients tended to speak more positively about what they had eaten and were less likely to discuss quantity. For examples of their statements see Box 12.1.

Box 12.1 Quotations found by Holden (20) in her study of cancer patients and their care givers. Examples of differences between patients and their care givers in reporting eating.

A 70-year-old patient said:
'I have been liking cold things, especially grapefruit juice, milk or ice cream.'

Meanwhile, her husband's comment was:

'She doesn't want more than a bite or two of food. She loves drink and small amounts of juice, not nearly enough. I make whatever she wants but she doesn't eat it.'

Many family members spoke about the amount of time and energy they spent on selecting and preparing food for the patient. Some referred to nutritional advice given to them at the time of diagnosis and seemed determined to still abide by those suggestions. Both patients and care givers often spoke with sadness about the lost opportunity of eating together (20).

Holden (20) found that all but one of the family members reported alterations in their own eating habits, for example eating more:

Oh yes, I've gained 30 pounds. I never cook anymore. I eat my main meal at work at noon and then I just snack at home. I'll eat a half gallon of ice cream in front of the TV . . . I eat like I did when I was a little girl. My mother would always feed me when I was anxious.

Family members were asked about their role as 'food preparer'. Their responses expressed anger, frustration, sadness, and fear, at the loss of this part of their relationship (see box 12.2).

Box 12.2. Quotations found by Holden in her study of cancer patients and their care givers (20).

Examples of care givers' responses to the importance of preparing food.

'I've always done the cooking and have loved it. Now it takes him two hours to eat what I finish in 15 minutes. I leave him sitting in front of the TV while I do what I have to do.'

'He [the patient] used to cook, too. We had some special recipes that we would make together. It just isn't any fun anymore. I feel so sad when I'm in the kitchen.'

'I understand that he can't eat but I do get angry when he won't try after I've worked so hard to fix it. I used to love to cook.

Examples of patients' responses.

'She worries too much. She tries to force me to eat when I don't want to. It is really a source of conflict and it is driving me nuts.'

'It shows that he cares, but sometimes I get angry because he keeps nagging at me.'

Family members are more concerned about eating than patients

In comparison with patients, family members frequently reported anorexia to be of greater concern than other problems. Patients cited other symptoms such as pain, breathing difficulties, weakness, draining wounds, fluid build up, fear of death, and fear of being alone as more important (20). Comparing the prospective views of patients with the later reports of bereaved carers, Cartwright and Seale (26) showed poor agreement for descriptions of 'loss of appetite'. The mean squared congruence for this symptom was 0.11 and the range in their study was 0.67 (best) to 0 (worst) (26). In Holden's (20) study, nine out of 14 patients (64%) indicated they appreciated their care givers' efforts, but four (28%) reported their care givers tried too hard and this had become a source of conflict and/or anger (see Box 12.2 for examples). When asked how they would like family members to respond to their anorexia, the vast majority (71%) of patients indicated that family members should be less assertive or should simply let them choose what and how much they wanted to eat (20).

Loss of control

Coping strategies, such as denial, may be adversely affected by cachexia, because patients become unable to ignore their altered body image. This may result in patients feeling increasingly out of control regarding their situation and thus increase fears and anxieties.

The affects of asthenia, such as tiredness, weakness, and poor concentration, may also make a patient feel unable to take part in family life and reduce their control over their lives.

PSYCHOLOGICAL CAUSES OF ANOREXIA AND CACHEXIA

In addition to the many physical causes (see Chapter 1), cancer anorexia and cachexia may have multiple psychological causes and, in particular, anorexia is a well-recognized symptom of anxiety, adjustment disorders, depression, other psychiatric disorders, and food aversions (see Table 12.1).

Appetite is extremely sensitive to mood changes (27, 28). Mood changes are common at the time of diagnosis or learning of a recurrence. Many patients note that along with signs of distress such as insomnia and poor concentration, they lose their appetite. Any loss of weight may frighten patients and their families into believing that the disease is progressing (see body size as a marker for disease above), resulting in increased anxiety. Later, fears of relapse may also result in overeating. In some cases, among women with breast cancer, weight gain has been a marked concern (29).

The differential diagnosis between major depression and a physical origin of anorexia can be very difficult (see Table 12.1). Anorexia and cachexia may be consequent to a physical pathology, but may result in a secondary depression about the condition, or the depression may be a prime contributor to the anorexia and subsequent weight loss.

Psychiatric disorders pre-exist in some individuals who develop cancer and this can complicate care and contribute to anorexia and cachexia. Anorexia nervosa, affective, schizophrenic, and other psychotic syndromes can result in altered food intake and weight loss.

Food aversions are commonly noted in cancer. Learned food aversions develop as a result of the association between a given food or foods and an unpleasant symptom such as nausea or vomiting. Changes can also occur secondary to the disease or its treatment, particularly radiotherapy to the head and neck regions, where there is an alteration in the taste thresholds to urea and glucose. Furthermore, DeWys (30) found that patients with cancer produced elevated levels of lactate, a metabolite known to cause nausea in normal volunteers. He suggested that cancer patients eating a normal amount of carbohydrate may develop nausea due to the increased levels of lactate and subsequently develop a learned response. Studies with animals suggest that tumour growth is associated with the development of strong aversions to the available diet. The aversions appear to play a causal role in the development of tumor-induced anorexia. The physiological consequences of tumor growth may act as an unconditioned stimulus/stimuli in taste-aversion conditioning (31).

Table 12.1 Psychological causes of anorexia–cachexia

Cause	Examples and relationship
Anxiety and adjustment disorders	Appetite is extremely sensitive to mood. Distress may present with poor concentration, insomnia, and loss of appetite. Subsequent loss of weight may cause more distress because this is interpreted as a deterioration. Fears of recurrence or deterioration can make the patient and carer become anxious about eating and attempts to increase food intake result in increased anxiety and lessened eating.
Depresssion	Anorexia is a cardinal symptom of depression; depression may also result from the anorexia–cachexia syndrome. In advancing disease both can be common. Symptoms of depression include inability to eat, no appetite, progressive weight loss, and sense of hopelessness. It is often difficult to distinguish these two symptoms.
Other psychiatric disorders	These can include anorexia nervosa, affective disorders, schizophrenic disorders, other psychotic disorders, personality disorders, and paranoia (for example, suspicion of piosoning)
Food aversion	Specific food aversions (dislike of particular foods, sometimes treatment-related).

MANAGEMENT

Psychotherapeutic, educational, and behavioural interventions for anorexia–cachexia

The use of psychological and behavioural interventions in cancer patients is increasing, in particular as recent studies have suggested that these may impact on the quality of life and survival. These techniques have been used to both reduce the anxiety and distress accompanying anorexia and depression and to relieve the symptoms either in combination with other therapies or by themselves.

Simple behavioral techniques, for example attention to the ambience around meals, having the family share the meal, serving a favorite wine or beer, adding home-like settings such as candles, are often advocated (27, 28). Avoiding strongly flavored foods, such as barbecued meats or fish and replacing these with blander foods such as cottage cheese or fruits is often recommended (27, 28). Although advocated, these techniques remain largely unevaluated in controlled trials. However, they are simple and inexpensive to try on a patient by patient basis and are supported by strongly positive case reports (27, 28). Attention to those situations which cause most distress is important.

Relaxation and hypnosis have been reported in descriptive (32) and randomized studies to have successfully lowered anxiety and relieved anorexia and nausea symptoms. Relaxation training and imagery were studied in 52 female and 30 male out-patients who were undergoing curative (73) or palliative (9) radiotherapy. Patients were assigned to a relaxation training condition as an adjunct to radiation or a control condition that entailed education and counselling along with the radiotherapy. Using pre- and post-tests of the Profile of Mood States, significant reductions were noted in the treatment group in tension, depression, anger, and fatigue. In contrast, the control group remained the same except in the case of depression and fatigue, which were exacerbated significantly (33). In a randomized study 55 cancer patients (mean age 59.6 years) assessed as nutritionally at risk were randomly assigned to one of four groups: nutritional suplementation, relaxation training, both nutritional supplementation and relaxation training, or neither nutritional supplementation nor relaxation training. Weight gain was greatest for the relaxation groups; the most severe loss occurred in the control group (34).

Short-term group psychotherapy appears promising, although to date the studies have considered general symptoms, rather than those specifically of anorexia and cachexia. In a randomized controlled trial of 48 cancer patients receiving radiotherapy, group psychotherapy was shown to reduce fatigue, anorexia, and emotional distress according to the Schedule for Affective Disorders and Schizophrenia (SADS) when compared with controls who received no psychotherapy after 4 weeks (35). Fawzy (37) studied the effects of a structured, short-term group psychiatric intervention, of 6 weekly visits of 1.5 hours each, in 66 adult post-surgical patients with malignant melanoma: 38 participated in the intervention and 28 served as controls. His intervention consisted of health education, stress management, illness-related problem-solving skills training, and psychological support. At 6 weeks, Profile of Mood States scores showed that the intervention group reported higher levels of vigour. At 6 month follow-up, the differences between the groups had increased. The intervention group showed significantly less depression-dejection, fatigue-inertia, confusion-bewilderment, and total mood disturbance and significantly more vigour-activity. These subjects continued to use significantly more active-behavioral and active-cognitive coping methods than controls (36). The intervention group also showed changes in natural killer cells. At 5–6 years after the intervention, controls showed a significantly higher rate of death than the intervention group. Fawzy (37) suggested that psychiatric intervention had a beneficial impact on the quality of life as well as the survival of cancer patients.

Psychological distress and psychiatric disorders accompanying anorexia–cachexia

Poor communication from doctors, nurses, and other staff remains one of the over-riding concerns of cancer patients (38–40). In anorexia–cachexia where the patient may be easily fatigued it is particularly important. Nutritional advice may be needed (41). In-depth discussion is often needed to identify the cause or causes of the problems and these may prove to be quite different from what one might expect. There are many factors interwoven: these may include the family, finances, spiritual needs, guilt, anger, fear of dying, or unrelieved physical symptoms. Multi-professional approaches appear to have better results than single professions (42, 43). The relevant chaplain or pastor and social worker can have important roles in supporting the anxious and frightened patient. A psychiatrist or psychologist will be needed for more complicated problems or to assess psychiatric morbidity such as depression or severe anxiety states.

The patient may employ a number of different defence mechanisms and coping strategies including the following:

1. Regression – becoming more child-like.

2. Denial – to blot out or ignore some realities.

3. Rationalization – providing an alternative everyday explanation for symptoms or feelings rather than the true one.

4. Intellectualization – becoming theoretical (often used by doctors and nurses in painful situations).

5. Projection – pushing the problem on to others.

6. Displacement – displacing emotional energy into other thoughts and activities.

7. Introjection – looking within oneself to find solutions.

8. Repression – unconscious suppression of painful memories.

9. Withdrawal and avoidance – withdrawing from and avoiding painful situations.

Understanding these mechanisms can help staff to explain and empathize with a patient's behavior. Each individual will have usually a number of these defence mechanisms and coping strategies. These are automatic and unconscious. It is only when the mechanisms are in excess that problems occur – for example, excessive introjection can result in self-blame, isolation, and depression; excessive projection can result in alienation of friends and family members or paranoid states, and excessive displacement can lead to complete exhaustion followed by severe depression or anxiety (2).

Some patients find comfort from living day to day for what pleasures, joys, and comforts can be achieved in that day, or by keeping a diary and recording their enjoyments, looking always for the positive uplifting events. In persistent fear and anxiety, in addition to psychological and supportive therapies, short-acting benzodiazepines or tranquilizers can be helpful, particularly if the patient has a chronic anxiety state and was already taking a small dose of these medications. Sedating antidepressants, such as amitriptyline and dothiepin, are increasingly used in anxiety states and imipramine is helpful if there are panic attacks (2).

Depression often goes undetected, partly because patients do not readily volunteer the symptoms and partly because it is often difficult to decide where natural sadness ends and depression begins (44). Too often it is assumed that depression is to be expected or is untreatable. Depression is usually characterized by a gradual onset of the following symptoms and signs:

(1) depressed mood or irritability;

(2) loss of interest and enjoyment;

(3) agitation or retardation;

(4) self-neglect or self-mutilation;

(5) cognitive triad – self is worthless, outside world meaningless, and future hopeless;

(6) diurnal mood swings (low mood in the morning);

(7) early morning wakening;

(8) change in behaviour – becoming indecisive, withdrawn, and arguing.

Often the physical symptoms of depression such as weight loss, anorexia, fatigue, and constipation are less useful for diagnosis because these may be present due to the terminal illness. Depression should also be distinguished from an adjustment disorder – a maladaptive reaction to a stress that occurs within 3 months and persists for no more than 3 months. In this the symptoms are less specific than those of depression and often fluctuate from day to day and in general the adjustment disorder will respond to psychological support (1).

Management should include the following:

(1) Consider any organic causes of depression, particularly drugs including some diuretics and antihypertensives, cimetidine, metoclopramide, methotrexate, and vinblastine and, if possible, stop or alter these.

(2) Emotional and psychological support and therapies.

(3) Antidepressant drugs (1, 2, 9).

CONCLUSIONS AND CLINICAL IMPLICATIONS

Psychological distress and psychiatric disorders are very common, and have been found in patients shortly after diagnosis and in advanced disease with prevalences in the ranges of 10–30% and 10–79%, respectively. Psychological distress and psychiatric disorders appear as common or more so among the family members of patients. Cachexia, anorexia, and asthenia can cause specific additional problems, in particular in body image, as a barometer of condition or a sign of impending death, and as a source of conflict between patients and their family members. Food preparation may be seen as an act of love and/or as essential for survival, and lowered food intake and weight loss causes enormous anxiety and conflict. Family members or care givers may be more concerned about anorexia than patients and their interpretation of events differ – family members remember what has not been eaten, and patients what has.

Diagnosis and treatment is complicated by the fact that, in addition to physical causes, cancer anorexia, and cachexia may have multiple psychological causes. In particular, anorexia is a well-recognized symptom of anxiety, adjustment disorders, depression, other psychiatric disorders, and food aversions. The differential diagnosis between major depression and a physical origin of anorexia can be very difficult. Anorexia and cachexia may be consequent to a physical pathology, but may result in a secondary depression about the condition, or the depression may be a prime contributor to the anorexia and subsequent weight loss.

The use of psychological and behavioral interventions in cancer patients is increasing: as recent studies have suggested that these may improve the quality of life and survival. These techniques have been used to both reduce the anxiety and distress accompanying anorexia and depression and to relieve the symptoms either in combination with other therapies or by themselves. Simple behavioral techniques, for example attention to the ambience around meals, having the family share the meal, are simple and cheap to try and are recommended, although their effectiveness is based largely on case reports. In conjunction, relaxation and hypnosis can successfully lower anxiety, relieve anorexia and nausea symptoms, and produce weight gain, and thus are well worth trying. Two randomized studies of short-term group psychotherapy also showed psychological and anorexia or fatigue benefits, although neither was targeted towards anorexia or cachexia. Discussion and treatment of any co-existing psychological or psychiatric disorder should also be provided. Effective communication with patients and their families is essential and is an important component of treatment.

In the future, studies are needed to assess the nature of concerns among patients and their families more accurately and to assess the comparative effectiveness of treatments, including the simple behavioral changes, relaxation therapy, hypnosis, and group therapy in the management of anorexia and cachexia.

REFERENCES

1. Cody M. Depression and the use of antidepressants in patients with cancer. Palliat Med 1990;4:271–8.
2. Hodgson G. Depression, sadness and anxiety. In: the management of terminal malignant disease, 3rd edn (ed. Saunders C, Sykes N). London: Edward Arnold; 102–30.
3. Hopwood P, Howell A, Maguire P. Psychiatric morbidity in patients with advanced cancer of the breast: prevalence measured by two self-rating questionnaires. Br J Cancer 1991;62(2):349–52.
4. Hughes J, Lee D. Depression among cancer patients admitted for hospice care. In: Psychosocial Oncology (ed. Watson M, Greer S, Thomas C). Oxford: Pergamon Press, 1988;193–6.
5. Vachon MLS, Lancee WJ, Ghardirian P, Adair WK. Final report on the needs of persons living with cancer in Quebec. Toronto: Canadian Cancer Society, 1991.
6. Vachon MLS, Lancee WJ, Conway B, Adair WK. Final report on the needs of persons living with cancer in Manitoba. Toronto: Canadian Cancer Society, 1990.

7. Kaye JM, Gracely EJ. Psychological distress in cancer patients and their spouses. J Cancer Educa 1993;8(1):47–52.

8. Vachon M. Emotional problems in palliative medicine: patient, family and professional. In: Oxford textbook of palliative medicine. (ed. Doyle D, Hanks GWC, MacDonald N). Oxford 1993;10:577–605.

9. Breitbart W, Passik SD. Psychiatric aspects of palliative care. In: Oxford textbook of palliative medicine. (ed. Doyle D, Hanks GWC). Oxford 1993;609–27.

10. Bruera E, MacMillan K, Hanson J, Kuehn N, MacDonald RN. A controlled trial of megestrol acetate pm appetite, caloric intake, nutritional status and other symptoms in patients with advanced caner. Cancer 1990;66:1279–82.

11. Schmoll E. Risks and benefits of various therapies for cancer anorexia. Oncology 1992;49(Suppl 2):43–5.

12. Loprinzi CL, Ellison NM, Goldberg RM, Michalak JC, Burch PA. Alleviation of cancer anorexia and cachexia: studies of the Mayo clinic and the North Central Cancer Treatment Group. Seminars Oncol 1990;17(6)(Suppl 9):8–12.

13. Hockley JM, Dunlop R, Davies RJ. Survey of distressing symptoms in dying patients and their families in hospital and the response to a symptom control team. BMJ 1988;296: 1715–17.

14. Bruera E. Fainsinger R. Clinical management of cachexia and anorexia. In: Oxford textbook of palliative medicine. (ed. Doyle D, Hanks GWC, MacDonald N). Oxford 1993;330–7.

15. Bruera E. Clinical management of anorexia and cachexia in patients with advanced cancer. Oncology 1992;49(Suppl 2):35–42.

16. Thomas CD, Freeman RJ. The body esteem scale: construct validity of the female subscales. J Person Assess 1990;54(1/2):204–12.

17. Keeton WP, Cash TF, Brown TA. Body image or body images? Comparative multi-dimensional assessment among college students. J Person Assess 1990; 54(1&2): 213–30.

18. Hopwood P. The assessment of body image in cancer patients. Eur J Cancer 1993;29(2):276–81.

19. Nerenz Dr, Leventhal H, Love RR, Ringer KE. Psychological aspects of cancer chemotherapy. Int Rev Appl Psychol 1984;33(4):521–9.

20. Holden CM. Anorexia in the terminally ill cancer patient: the emotional impact on the patient and family. Hospice J 1991;7(3):73–84.

21. DeWys WD, Begg C, Lavin PT *et al.* Prognostic effective of weight loss prior to chemotherapy in cancer patients. Am J Med 1980;69:491–7.

22. Stanley KE. Prognostic factors for survival in patients with inoperable lung cancer. J Natl Cancer Inst 1980;65:484–8.

23. Bruera E, Miller MKN, MacEachern T *et al.* Estimate of survival of patients admitted to a palliative care unit: a prospective study. J Pain Symptom Manage 1992;7(2):82–6.

24. Dixon CE, Emery AW Jr, Hurley RS. Nutrition in cancer patients with a limited life expectancy. Am J Hospice Care 1985;2(3):27–33.

25. Donovan MI, Pierce SG. Cancer care nursing. New York: Appleton-Century-Crofts, 1976.

26. Cartwright A, Seale C. The natural history of a survey: an account of the methodological issues encountered in a study of life before death. London: King Edwards Hospital Fund, 1990.

27. Lesko LM. Psychological issues in the diagnosis and management of cancer cachexia and anorexia. Nutrition 1989;5(2):114–16.

28. Lesko LM. Anorexia. Special issues in the psychological management of cancer. In: Handbook of psycho-oncology: psychological care of the patient with cancer (ed. Holland JC, Rowland JH). New York: Oxford University Press, 1989; 434–42.

29. Monnin S, Schiller MR, Saches L, Smith A. Nutrition concerns of women with breast cancer. J Cancer Educat 1993;8(1):63–9.

30. DeWys WD. Pathophysiology of cancer cachexia. Current understanding and areas for future research. Cancer Res 1982;42:721s.
31. Bernstein IL. Learning food aversions in the progression of cancer and its treatment. Ann NY Acad Sci 1985;443:365–80.
32. Kaye JM. Use of hypnosis in the treatment of cancer patients. J Psychosoc Oncol 1987;5(2):11–22.
33. Decker TW, Cline–Elsen J, Gallagher M. Relaxation therapy as an adjunct in radiation oncology. J Clin Psychol 1992;48(3):388–93.
34. Dixon J. Effect of nursing interventions on nutritional and performance status in cancer patients. Nursing Res 1984;33(6):330–5.
35. Forester B, Kornfeld DS, Fleiss JL, Thompson S. Group psychotherapy during radiotherapy: effects on emotional and physical distress. Am J Psychiat 1993; 150(11):1700–6.
36. Fawzy FL, Cousins N, Fawzy NW et al. A structured psychiatric intervention for cancer patients: I. Changes over time in methods of coping and affective disturbance. Arch Gen Psychiat 1990;47(8):720–5.
37. Fawzy FI. The benefits of a short-term group intervention for cancer patients. Advances 1994;10(2):17–19.
38. Higginson I, Wade A, McCarthy M. Palliative care: views of patients and their families. BMJ 1990;301:277–81.
39. Maguire P, Faulkner A. Communicating with cancer patients: 1. Handling bad news and difficult questions. BMJ 1988;297:907–9.
40. Maguire P, Faulkner A. Communicating with cancer patients: 2. Handling uncertainty, collusion and denial. BMJ 1988;297:972–4.
41. Tchekmedyian NS, Zahyna D, Halpert C et al. Clinical aspects of nutrition in advanced cancer. Oncology 1992;49(Suppl 2):3–7.
42. Jones RVH. Teams and terminal cancer at home: do patients and carers benefit? J Interprofession Care 1993;7(3):239–44.
43. Vachon MLS. Counselling and psychotherapy in palliative/hospice care: a review. Palliat Med 1988;2:36–50.
44. Maguire P. Monitoring the quality of life in cancer patients and their relatives. In: Cancer: assessment and monitoring. (ed. Symington T, Williams AE, McVie JG). London: Churchill Livingstone, 1980;40–52.

Practical concepts for clinicians

Irene Higginson and Eduardo Bruera

INTRODUCTION

In previous chapters we have discussed, in depth, a number of issues related to the cachexia–anorexia complex. This present chapter aims to summarize those aspects that are particularly relevant to practising clinicians. Instead of traditional references, we refer the reader to the specific chapter where each subject is discussed in more depth.

EPIDEMIOLOGY

The cachexia–anorexia syndrome is now well recognized and defined. It is found in over 50% and in some studies up to 90% of cancer patients: this varies depending on the population included. Cachexia is more common in patients with advanced disease than those in early stages of illness, and among patients with solid tumours, except for breast cancer, compared with haematological malignancies. Older patients may also be somewhat less likely to experience anorexia than younger patients. The high prevalence of this syndrome and the distress it causes patients and families means that it is an important symptom for all doctors, nurses, and other professionals working with cancer patients. In research terms there is much to be done in separating symptoms due to this syndrome from other causes of weight loss and loss of appetite, and on the development of staging systems and effective therapeutic alternatives.

PRESENTATION AND AETIOLOGY

Although there is a broad spectrum of clinical presentations, almost all patients suffering from the cachexia–anorexia syndrome exhibit weight loss, loss of appetite, weakness, and lassitude. This clinical picture results from progessive wasting of structural protein and energy stores and inevitably leads to a global decline in functioning. As Chapter 1 describes, early hopes that a single cachexic mediator would be identified have given way to the belief that cachexia arises from a complex interaction between the cancer and the host. These can include tumour aspects such as cytokine production, the release of lipid mobilizing factors, mechanical obstruction, or substrate consumption. Within the patient there may be increased resting energy expenditure, alterations in intermediary metabolism, cytokine production by host macrophages and autonomic dysfunction such as reduced gastric emptying. Treatment-related effects such as nausea, stomatitis, mucositis, xerostomia, fatigue, pain or ileus as a result of chemotherapy, radiotherapy or surgery may also contribute. Psychological factors may have a role as a result of learned food aversions, alterations in taste perception or stress. However, in spite of the complexity of these factors and the interplay between tumour and host, these networks appear to rely on initiating signal cytokines, which in turn lead to the amplification of other cytokines or mediators. In the future, if these primary signalling molecules and their receptors can be identified they may provide an opportunity to circumvent many of the devastating effects of cachexia–anorexia.

ASSOCIATED SYMPTOMS

Symptoms such as chronic nausea, asthenia (fatigue, easy tiring, weakness, and mental fatigue), and lesions of the oral cavity, in particular fungal infections including candidiasis, herpetic infections, ulcers, stomatitis, xerostomia (mouth dryness), taste alteration, and tumours within the mouth, are all common alongside the cachexia–anorexia syndrome. Although these symptoms can present independently from cachexia–anorexia, in many patients they develop in parallel. Often one symptom may contribute to the development of another. Chronic nausea and oral complications should be treated actively and guidance in the assessment, diagnosis, and management of these symptoms and their various aetiologies is given in Chapters 2 and 3, respectively.

Cachexia–anorexia must be considered within the holistic context of the patient and his or her family members or carers. Just as total pain has been well recognized for many years and includes physical, emotional, social, and spiritual concepts so the anorexia–cachexia syndrome has physical, emotional, social, and spiritual components. The syndrome interacts with many of the other common symptoms found in cancer such as pain, dyspnoea, constipation, and psychosocial and spiritual aspects such as the patient and family's emotional reaction, their social resources including family status, financial situation, and physical environment. Chapter 11 provides six guidelines for comprehensive assessment which includes the assessment of anorexia–cachexia. These include symptom evaluation and investigation review, assessment of symptom and disease impact, diagnostic investigations and specific assessments, assessment of symptom pathophysiology, global assessment, and multimodality therapeutic plan.

ASSESSMENT OF NUTRITIONAL STATE, INTAKE, AND APPETITE

Nutritional state is usually evaluated with a combination of clinical assessment and anthropometric tests such as body weight, skin fold thickness, and mid arm circumference. These are cheap, quick, and simple tests which do not require extensive equipment and make them particularly useful for patients suffering advancing cancer. Grip strength as measured by a dynamometer is increasing in use and may be of value. A number of laboratory tests are available, such as the measurement of short half-life protein and analysis of urinary metabolites, but many of these are of limited value among cancer patients because of the chronic nature of malnutrition. Immunological tests are not useful because of the effects of cancer or the therapies on lymphocyte activity. Serum albumin is one of the most common parameters used because of its low cost and accuracy in the absence of nephropathy or liver failure.

Other methods to assess nutritional status tend to be used mainly in research settings: these include infra-red interactions, where the reflection absorption or transmission of infra-red light is recorded; and bioimpedance resistance and electroconductivity, which measure the resistance of the body to the flow of alternating electrical current. Bioelective impedance may be of special interest in the future because of its ability to determine total body water and total body lean mass. Its non-invasive nature and low cost allow for repeated assessment during therapy. Computer tomography, magnetic resonance imaging (MRI), and ultrasound imaging may also have a role in research studies.

Calorie intake is much more difficult to assess and relies on dietary records of either weighted or estimated food quantities; recall questionnaires; prospective recording; or evaluation by a third person. Appetite can be assessed fairly simply using visual analogue scales or patient questionnaires.

In a clinical setting nutritional status and appetite can be assessed using simple techniques and recordings and we would recommend that these are developed within the clinical setting. While the diagnosis of malnutrition can be made easily with the medical history and physical exam, the follow-up of changes over time may be impossible unless nutritional assessment takes place. In research studies and particularly in the evaluation of drugs, assessment of calorific intake and a nutritional status need to be undertaken more rigorously.

PSYCHOLOGICAL DIMENSIONS

Psychological distress and psychiatric disorders are common among cancer patients and have been found with prevalence ranging from 10 to 79% of patients depending upon the group studied. These problems are also as common or more so among the family members. The cachexia–anorexia syndrome can cause specific and additional psychological problems. Body image may be disturbed. Weight loss may be seen as a barometer of the condition or as a sign of impending death and eating may become a source of conflict between the patients and their family members. The preparation of food is often seen as an act of love and/or as essential for survival and so reduced food intake and weight loss can cause enormous anxiety and conflict within the family. Studies have suggested that family members may be more concerned about the anorexia–cachexia than patients themselves and each interprets events differently: family members tend to remember what hasn't been eaten, patients remember what was eaten.

Anorexia and cachexia may also have multiple psychological causes and these must be considered in the differential diagnosis. Anorexia is a well recognized symptom of anxiety, adjustment disorders, depression, other psychiatric disorders, and food aversions and the differential diagnosis between major depression and a physical origin of anorexia can be very difficult. These disorders may become interrelated in that anorexia and cachexia may result in secondary depression about the condition or, alternatively, depression may be the prime contributor to anorexia and subsequent weight loss.

REHYDRATION AND NUTRITIONAL SUPPORT: TREATMENT AND ETHICS

The ethical considerations and indications for either hydration or enteral or parenteral nutrition in patients with advanced cancer are complex and much of the data in the literature are descriptive rather than evaluative. Review of the literature in Chapter 7 on the effects of dehydration suggests that while some dying patients do not suffer any ill effects from dehydration there may be others who manifest symptoms, such as confusion or opioid toxicity, which may be alleviated by hydration.

Hypodermoclysis is the infusion of fluids into the subcutaneous space. This method was used widely in clinical practice in the 1940s and 50s but then fell from popularity. However, it is re-emerging as a method which is potentially useful in palliative care especially among patients with very advanced disease; in patients with earlier stages of disease and who are dehydrated intravenous hydration is the most common evaluated method.

Enteral and parenteral nutrition, as discussed in Chapter 8, appear to be of much less value. There are no clear suggestions from this review that nutritional support effectively improves the complications of malnutrition in cancer patients. Although enteral nutrition and total parenteral nutrition have been shown to reverse malnutrition partially, they do not combat cancer and any lasting benefit of nutritional therapy has always been related to the effectiveness of antineoplastic treatment. A step-wise approach to decision making which defines the clinical condition, the expected survival, assesses the hydration and nutritional state, the symptoms, nutritional intake, psychological attitude, gut functions, and the social, cultural, and scientific background of the patient could be a useful model for making decisions within clinical practice.

There are certain cancer patients who may benefit from nutritional support, particularly if they are malnourished and undergoing antineoplastic treatments with high nutritional morbidities or if they are unable to swallow for some reason but have normal appetite and good performance status. In contrast, patients in a terminal stage of cancer with malignant bowel obstruction and confined to bed may find nutritional support increases their distress. Parenteral nutrition has a complication rate of 15% and high costs, and is no longer considered different from and/or superior to enteral nutrition in reversing malnutrition. Therefore enteral feeding of cancer patients is favoured when it is possible and not contraindicated. Chapter 10 provides further guidance to the role of enteral tubes, gastrostomy, and jejunostomy for feeding and venting purposes in advanced cancer. This chapter also provides a guide to decision making when considering gastric feeding, which may be of extra value in earlier stages of disease.

CLINICAL GUIDELINES

The clinical management of cachexia in cancer patients should first concentrate on simple solutions such as maximizing oral intake by allowing the patient flexibility in the type, quantity, and timing of the food and by the management of associated nausea, oral lesions, or other symptoms. Simple behavioral techniques, for example attending to the ambience around meals, having the family share the meal if they wish, and exploring concerns about the eating with both a family member and the patient to relieve anxiety and remove conflict, may be very helpful. Effective communication with the patient and the family will be essential to achieve this and assess the nature of the problem and appropriate treatment.

Artificial nutrition, including parenteral and enteral nutrition may be indicated in a very small proportion of advanced cancer patients. As discussed above, these techniques should be considered in the context of a cost-benefit equation on an individualized basis.

The main purpose of the pharmacological treatment of cachexia is to counteract its two main symptoms, anorexia, and chronic nausea. Ideally, an improvement in muscle metabolism and asthenia could also be goals of the treatment, but it remains to be determined whether new approaches can achieve this.

Progestational drugs have received the most attention during the recent years. Megestrol acetate has been found to improve appetite, food intake, and nutritional status in both cancer and AIDS patients. Medroxyprogesterone acetate has been found to produce a similar result. Doses ranging between 480 and 960 mg per day appear to be the most effective in producing objective and subjective improvement. The beneficial effects of these drugs are probably not related to the increase in oral intake, since a similar improvement has not been observed with aggressive enteral and parenteral nutrition. More likely, these drugs act on a more fundamental abnormality on some of the metabolic pathways and the improvement in appetite, food intake, and fatigue may be a result of a change in the catabolic state rather than the cause of the improvement. A similar improvement in appetite, food intake, and energy is observed in patients as a result of antibiotic therapy for an acute infection or after the immediate post-operative period. In patients in whom profound anorexia is the main manifestation of cachexia, megestrol acetate will be useful if the patient is expected to survive for weeks to months, because of its effects on both appetite and nutritional status.

A number of controlled trials have found that corticosteroids are able to improve appetite, sensation of well-being, and energy in advanced cancer patients. Unfortunately, both food intake and nutritional status have not been found to improve significantly, and the overall duration of the response is short, usually measured in weeks. In addition, prolonged corticosteroid treatment has been associated with weakness, delirium, osteoporosis, and immunosuppression, all of which are commonly present in advanced cancer. The optimal type, dose, and route of administration of corticosteroids has not been established. However, in patients with a short expected survival or those who have problems tolerating progestational drugs, a brief course of corticosteroids may be useful. These drugs can be administered both orally and subcutaneously and, in addition to stimulating appetite, they have effects on nausea, pain, and asthenia. While progestational agents are able to increase the patient's caloric intake and improve nutritional status, however, the effects of corticosteroids are, as discussed above, short lasting and merely symptomatic. Other pharmacological treatments are currently being investigated. However, they have received insufficient evaluation to be recommended in clinical practice.

Psychological and behavioral interventions in cancer are increasing in use and recent studies have suggested that some of these may affect quality of life and survival. Evaluations of relaxation, hypnosis, and short-term group psychotherapy have suggested some benefit in anorexia and fatigue, although the population most likely to benefit from these interventions has not yet been established.

In the future, a better understanding of the host and tumour mediators of cachexia may lead to more focused pharmacological interventions to relieve these symptoms. Comparative evaluations of psychological and behavioral interventions may also indicate which of these are or are not helpful in improving this syndrome, to what extent and for which patients.

Index

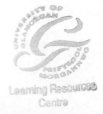